W9-AUD-541

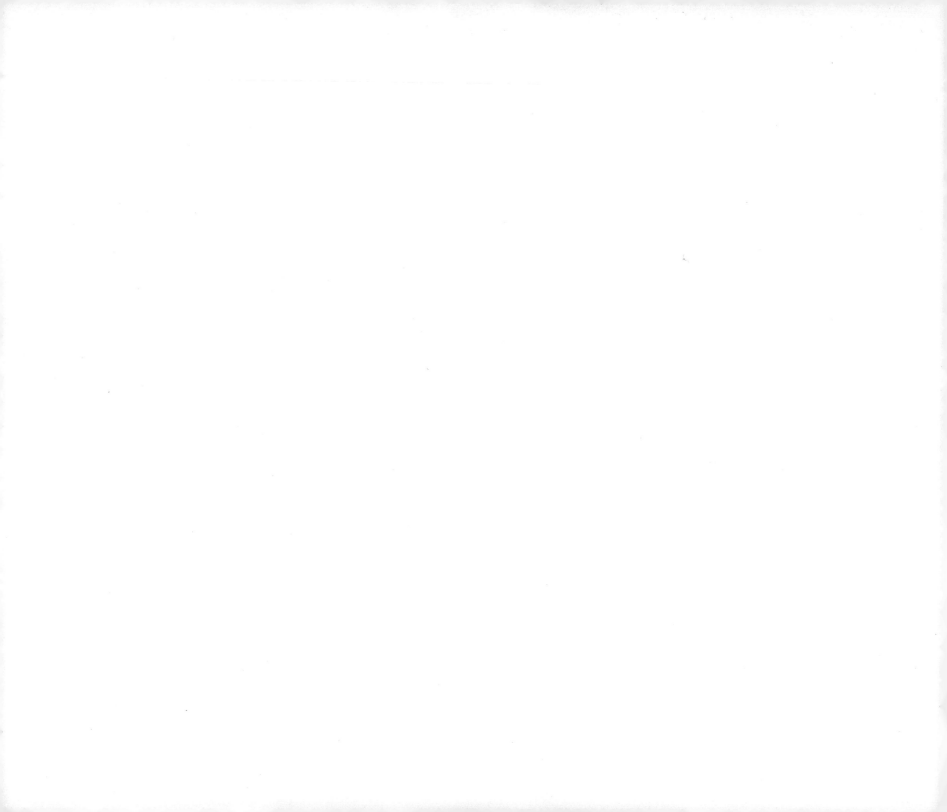

Locomotion

Overleaf *The universal contrast: Man versus*
Nature, between Mount Fuji and the Bullet
Train – one of the first lines in Japan took pilgrims
to the holy mountain.

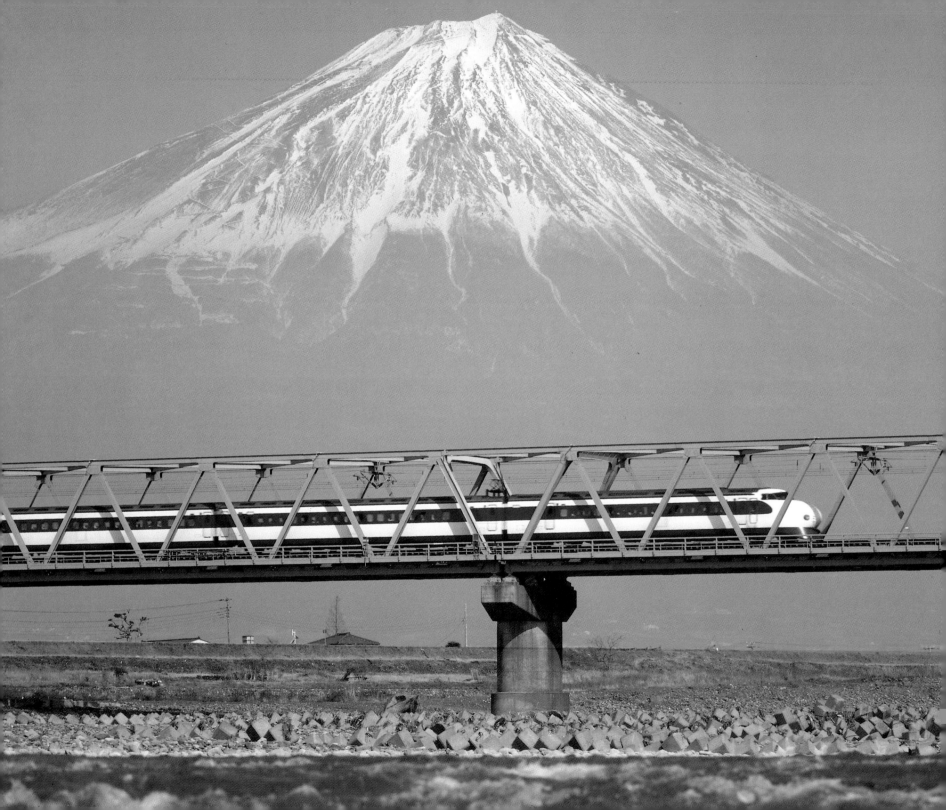

·LOCOMOTION·

THE RAILWAY REVOLUTION

Nicholas Faith

BBC Books

Published by BBC Books,
a division of BBC Enterprises Limited,
Woodlands, 80 Wood Lane, London W12 0TT

First published 1993
© Nicholas Faith 1993
The moral rights of the author have been asserted
ISBN 0 563 36740 7
Designed by Tim Higgins
Set in Adobe Stone Serif by Selwood Systems,
Midsomer Norton
Printed and bound in Great Britain
by Butler & Tanner Ltd, Frome and London
Colour separations by Technik Ltd, Berkhamsted
Jacket printed by Lawrence Allen Ltd,
Weston-super-Mare

Acknowledgements

This book was originally designed to accompany the series of the same name on BBC2, but for various reasons the text strayed rather from the series. So I am particularly grateful to all those involved for their patience at my erring ways.

Those involved in the series – especially the Executive Producer Peter Grimsdale – were extraordinarily helpful, and thanks are also due to Peter Bate, Tim Copestake, Elizabeth Dobson, Vivian Ducat, Lisbet Heath, Norma Howson, Tim Jordan, Gerald Lorenz, Val Mitchell, Isabel Pritchard, Lawrence Simanowitz, Tuppence Stone and Duncan Thomson.

BBC Books turned out to be exemplary publishers. Sheila Ableman was kindly but firm, as befits a boss, Julian Flanders infinitely patient in the tradition of the best editors, and David Cottingham did an astonishing job in finding visual material of a variety and quality which rendered me almost speechless.

Thank you.

Nicholas Faith 1993

Picture Credits

BBC Books would like to thank the following for providing photographs and for permission to reproduce copyright material. While every effort has been made to trace and acknowledge all copyright holders, we would like to apologize should there have been any errors or omissions:

Page 2 Tony Stone Worldwide; **6** Courtesy Darlington Museum; **9** Mary Evans Picture Library; **10** National Railway Museum; **11** Steve Dunwell/Image Bank; **12** Hulton Deutsch Collection; **14** Giuliano Colliva/Image Bank; **15** Robert Harding Picture Library; **18–19** Bridgeman Art Library; **21 and 22** National Railway Museum; **23** Bridgeman Art Library; **24** Hulton Deutsch Collection; **25** Mary Evans Picture Library; **26** Steve McCurry/Magnum; **30** British Museum, Dept of Japanese Antiquities; **31** Bridgeman Art Library; **34–35** Alan Becker/Image Bank; **36** Library of Congress; **37** Smithsonian Institute, Washington; **39** Robert Harding Picture Library; **41** Leicestershire Museum; **42** Victoria and Albert Museum; **43** National Railway Museum; **44** Photo Researchers, Inc; **49** Victoria and Albert Museum; **50** British Library, India Office Library; **52–53** J. M. Jarvis/Zefa; **56** Mary Evans Picture Library; **57** L. Allan Cash; **58** Library of Congress;

59 Hulton Deutsch Collection; **60** Punch Publications Ltd; **64** Popperfoto; **65** National Railway Museum; **66** Robert Harding Picture Library; **68** K. Goebel/Zefa; **69** Mary Evans Picture Library; **72** Ballantyne/Zefa; **75** Illustrated London News; **76–77** Randy Taylor/Katz Pictures; **79** Imperial War Museum; **82** Library of Congress/Brady Collection; **84** Illustrated London News; **85** Gysenbergh/Gamma/Frank Spooner Pictures; **87** Hulton Deutsch Collection; **88 and 89** Colin Garratt/Milepost 92½; **93** National Railway Museum; **94 and 95** Hulton Deutsch Collection; **97** Mary Evans Picture Library; **98** E. T. Archive; **100 and 101** Steve McCurry/Magnum; **103** Popperfoto; **104** Hutchison Library; **109** Robert Francis/South American Pictures; **110** Tony Morrison/South American Pictures; **112** Anthony J. Lambert Collection; **113** Tony Gervis/Robert Harding Picture Library; **117** Colin Garratt/Milepost 92½; **120** Hiroji Kubota/Magnum; **122–123** Uthoff/Image Bank; **124** Union Pacific Railroad Collection; **125 (both)** Hulton Deutsch Collection; **126 and 127** Zefa; **131** Anthony J. Lambert Collection; **133** Nebraska State Historical Society; **134** Library of Congress; **139** Tony Stone Worldwide/Click Chicago; **143** Birmingham Museums and Art Gallery; **145** National Railway Museum; **146** Library of Congress; **148** Victoria and Albert Museum;

149 Gruyaert/Magnum; **151** Popperfoto; **152** Robert Harding Picture Library; **154** Hulton Deutsch Collection; **156** Illustrated London News; **157** Rolf Richardson/Robert Harding Picture Library; **158** Illustrated London News; **160** Errington/Hutchison Library; **164** Images Colour Library; **168** Hutchison Library; **170** Zefa; **171 (right)** John Egan/Hutchison Library; **172** Popperfoto; **174 (left)** RIBA; **175** British Library, India Office Library; **177** Hulton Deutsch Collection; **178** Achim Sperber/Image Bank; **181** British Museum, Dept of Japanese Antiquities; **183** Robert Harding Picture Library; **185** Kobal Collection; **186** National Gallery, London; **187 (left)** Hulton Deutsch Collection; **187 (right)** Bridgeman Art Library; **190** National Railway Museum; **191** Bridgeman Art Library/Aberdeen Art Gallery and Museum; **196, 197, 199 and 200** Kobal Collection; **202** Patrick Whitehouse; **206–207** Robert Harding Picture Library; **209** Camera Press; **210** Bradshaw/Saba/Katz Pictures; **211** Bridgeman Art Library; **214** J. Allan Cash; **215** Images Colour Library; **219** Zachmann/Magnum; **220** AISA Archivo Iconografico; **223** Tony Stone Worldwide; **224** Richard Kalvar/Magnum; **226** Anthony J. Lambert Collection; **230** Courtesy CSX; **234** Courtesy Voyages Jules Verne/Serenissima Travel; **235** Q A Photos.

Contents

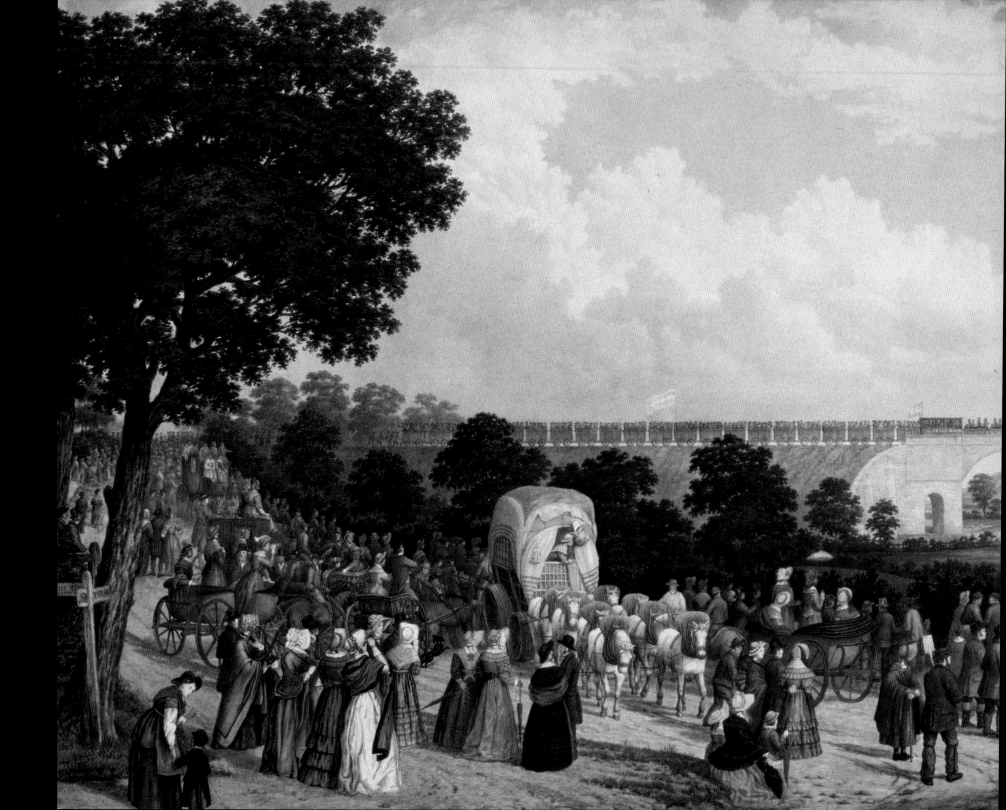

Introduction

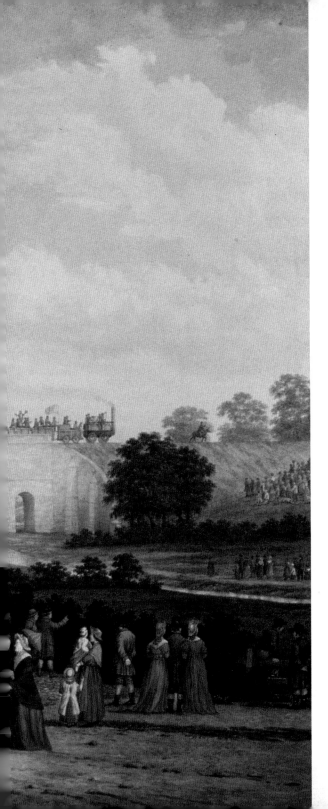

It seems to me as if this railway were the one typical achievement of the age in which we live, as if it brought together into one plot all the ends of the world and all the degrees of social rank and offered to some great writer the busiest, the most extended, and the most varied subject for an enduring literary work. If it be romance, if it be contrast, if it be heroism that we require, what was Troy town to this?

*I*n his travel notes (collected as *The Amateur Emigrant*) Robert Louis Stevenson posed a challenge, to which no single author, however talented, could ever adequately respond. For, in the words of the old newspaper slogan, 'all human life is here', clustered along the tracks, on the footplate, in the open carriages and closed compartments of the trains themselves, riding the rails, working for the railways, lurking in the stations.

The effects of the railways on society are too universal and long-lasting to be compressed within a single volume. Like some many-headed Hindu god they contain life and death, creation and destruction, squalor and magnificence. All I can do is to sketch some of the more interesting aspects, to provide my readers with food for thought, to enable them to look more closely, not so much at the railways they use, as at the townscape and landscape around them, and to detect their still all-pervasive influence.

The railway was the first, the most universal and the most dramatic mechanical intrusion into the lives of peoples and nations, the first of the technical revolutions

John Dobbin's depiction of the opening of the Stockton to Darlington Railway in 1825 over-romanticizes the first intrusion of the mechanical monster into a rural idyll.

which created the world as we know it today. It was also the most fundamental, the most long-lasting, for it was the first time that man, through sheer mechanical ingenuity, had been able to impose his will on nature and thus transform his relationship with nature. Yet (and this, perversely, is a recurrent theme running through this book) even this, the first such innovation, could not dramatically alter human nature and, as we shall see, the railways carried with them their own limitations. Their power was neither total nor infinite.

Curiously, and notably unlike later major inventions which have transformed man's relationship with nature – from the internal combustion engine, through radio to television, the jet engine, the computer and the silicon chip – the actual innovations required to develop a steam locomotive riding on iron wheels on an iron road were not in themselves dramatic or revolutionary. For centuries miners had used rails of wood or iron to carry horse-drawn wagon-loads of coal from their pits to the nearest navigable water. For half a century before the first steam-powered railway opened in 1825 from Stockton to Darlington, steam engines had been at work in the very same mines which used railways. And as early as 1803 Richard Trevithick had already used high-pressure steam engines to haul wagons in the tin mines in Cornwall.

But George Stephenson, still rightly regarded as the father of the railways, possessed two great advantages denied to Trevithick and other putative parent figures: enough capital, and a series of improvements both in the iron used for the rails and in their form – for the flanged wheel developed in the North-East running on iron rails wastes less energy than any other combination. Nevertheless it took a very particular type of genius to develop the system, to install it and above all to sell it to hard-headed financiers and a sceptical public. This was the genius not of a scientist or inventor, nor even a great engineer – Stephenson had no training and was virtually uneducated – but of a man of character, of implacable will-power, combined with a vision of the future. Perhaps the best tribute came, not from the British, for whom he was a controversial figure, but from the Italians when they set up a plaque at Poggibonsi station near Florence: *A la gloria imperitura di Giorgio Stephenson. I ferroviarii di Poggibonsi* (To the imperishable glory of George Stephenson, from the railwaymen of Poggibonsi).

His combination of steam power and railways would not have been possible in any other corner of Britain (and was inconceivable anywhere else in the world). For at the time the north-east of England had the same combination of technical innovation backed by venture capital found, say, in California's Silicon Valley in the age of the micro-chip. In Professor Jack Simmons' words, Stephenson, his son Robert, and Isambard Kingdom Brunel, the three giants of the first decades of the Age of Steam, founded 'a school: a school of practice and experience that quickly permeated the whole island and reached out across the world.'

An alliance between the glorified blacksmith and enterprising and innovative local capitalists created the Stockton and Darlington, the first railway worked primarily by steam power. This radical initiative set the pace for developments which, within half a century, had changed the face of the world – and of man's expectations – for ever.

For the railway system Stephenson assembled has proved immensely durable, seemingly eternal. While the two other great mechanical innovations of the nineteenth century, the electric telegraph and the steamship, have been largely overtaken (by radio waves and by aeroplanes respectively), the railways' future has never seemed more promising. For a generation after 1945 they seemed to be at the mercy of cars, lorries and buses powered by internal combustion engines. But the limitations of over-reliance on road transport have become only too apparent over the past two decades, the cost in human, environmental and even efficiency terms increasing exponentially. At the same time the railways have demonstrated that they can safely carry passengers for long distances at an average speed of over 100 mph (160 kph) on the historic lines laid down in the nineteenth century, and double that speed on the increasing number of new ones being built – and planned.

Like the original impact, the resulting renaissance, analysed in Chapter 10, is universal, the only differences being that the new railwaymen are starting from an existing base, and that the spread is even faster. The first special ultra-fast new line was opened in Japan in 1964, and the first in Europe, from Paris to Lyon, in 1983. Yet within a decade every country in Europe has evolved similar plans, and in many cases – notably in Spain, Germany and Italy – the rails are actually being laid. In a few years' time the emerging

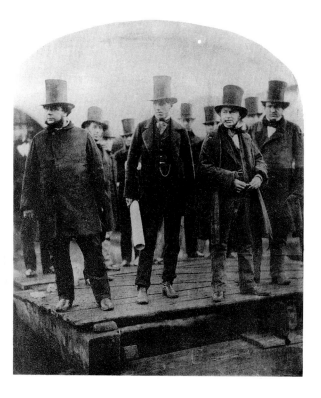

Isambard Kingdom Brunel (second from right) *chewing the inevitable cigar at the attempted launch of the ship the* Great Eastern *in 1857.*

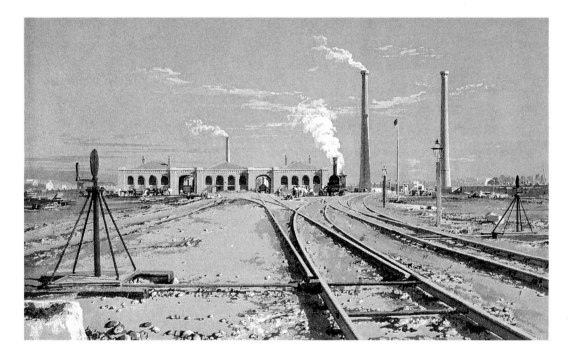

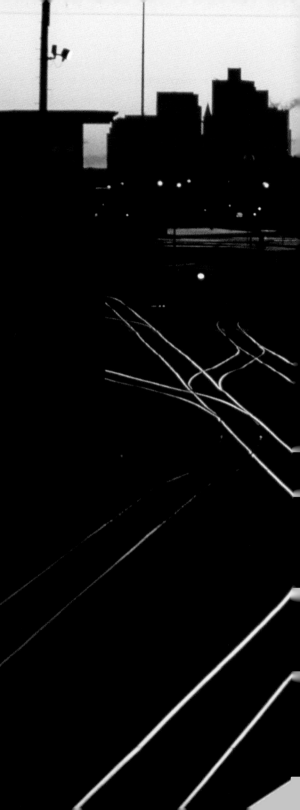

Above *One of the first ever pictorial representations of the railways. Thomas Bourne based his famous prints on wash drawings like this – of the locomotive engine house at Camden Town in London.*

Right *The tracks in this marshalling yard look like roots nourishing the skyscrapers of downtown Boston, emphasising the contrast between homely London and the scale of metropolitan America.*

pan-European network of new lines will pose a challenge to the aeroplane for many routes of less than 800 km (500 miles) – from London to Paris and Brussels, from Paris to Cologne and Amsterdam, from Rome to Turin and Milan. Yet all these new trains will be using the same principles as those established by George Stephenson in the third decade of the nineteenth century: they will be composed of engines and carriages with steel wheels running on steel rails 143.5 cm (4 ft 8½ in) apart, and they will be propelled by an electric motor of the type first built by Dr Siemens over a century ago.

Even today – indeed especially and increasingly today – the state of a country's railways reflects the state of the country itself. In the words of Paul Theroux, most

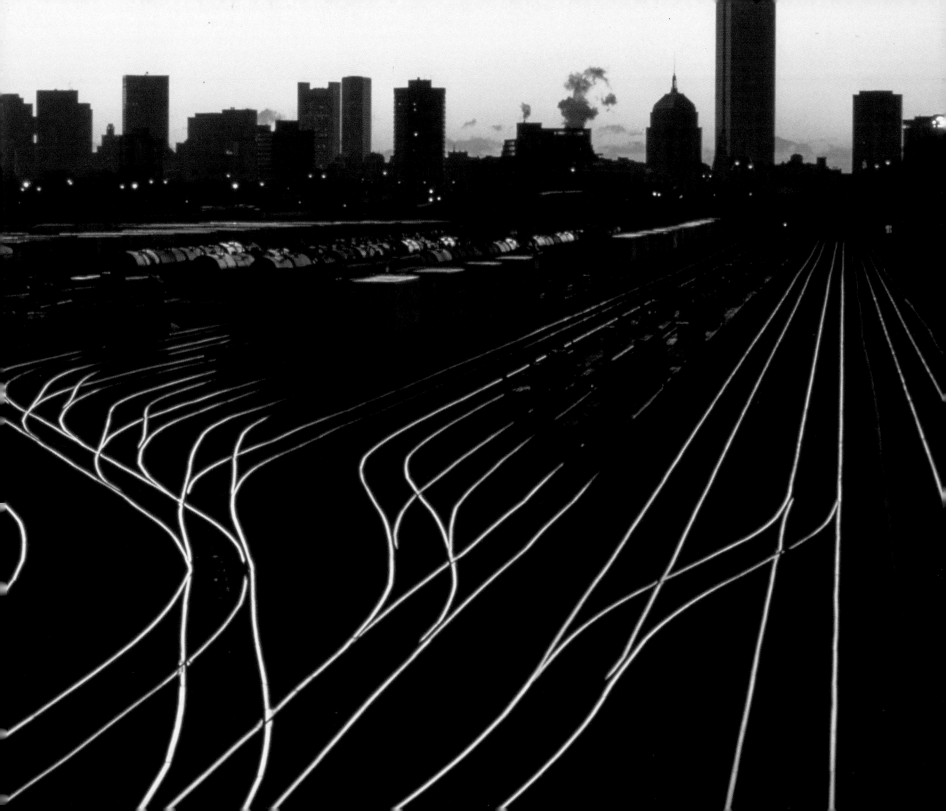

perceptive of rail travellers, 'The seedy, distressed country has seedy, distressed railway trains, the proud, efficient nation is similarly reflected in its rolling stock.' Theroux singles out Japan, whose industrial miracle was first signalled by the opening of the New Tokaido line in 1964. The Japanese would agree. Ever since they opened their country to Western influences they have measured their progress through their steadily-increasing success in operating railways and building locomotives. Similarly the renewed mechanical daring of the French is signalled by the TGV – and the relative decline of Anglo-Saxon economies by the decline of Canada's railways, the belated attempts by the Americans to revive theirs and the grudging attitude of the British towards investment in theirs.

*F*or all the novelty of rail, the earliest travellers immediately understood its magic and its possibilities. The first account we have of rail travel and its creator remains, in my eyes, the most perfect, the dawn of a new age captured, as was only proper, by someone young. Fanny Kemble, a member of the most distinguished theatrical family of the day, was one of the first passengers carried by George Stephenson on the *Rocket* during the trials of the locomotive before the opening of the Liverpool & Manchester railway. The description, by a girl of enchanting wit and beauty, perfectly captures a unique moment when the world was young and full of magic. George Stephenson, always canny, ever aware of the advantages of favourable publicity, had chosen well. She found him a man

> ... of an immense constructiveness ... a man of from fifty to fifty-five years of age; his face is fine, though careworn, and bears an expression of deep thoughtfulness; his mode of explaining his ideas is peculiar and very original, striking and forcible; and although his accent indicates strongly his north-country birth, his language has not the slightest touch of vulgarity or coarseness. He has certainly turned my head.

To her the engine was a 'steam-horse' (the Americans habitually referred to a locomotive as the 'Iron Horse'), a 'snorting little animal which I felt rather inclined to pat.' Because the beast was

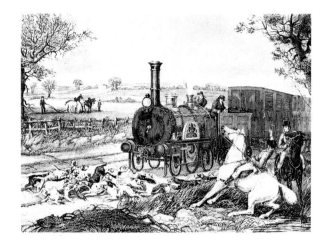

As late as 1855 Henry Alken was portraying the great fear of the British aristocracy, that the railways would interfere with their fox-hunting.

... ill-adapted for going up and down hill, the road was kept at a certain level, and appeared, sometimes to sink below the surface of the earth and sometimes to rise above it. ... You can't imagine how strange it seemed to be journeying on thus, without any visible cause of progress other than the magical machine, with its flying white breath and rhythmical, unvarying pace, between these rocky walls, which are already clothed with moss and ferns and grasses ... when I closed my eyes the sensation of flying was quite delightful and strange beyond description; yet strange as it was, I had a perfect sense of security, and not the slightest fear ... I felt as if no fairy tale was ever half so wonderful as what I saw.

Fanny Kemble's feelings were not universally shared. At 20 mph (32 kph) Thomas Creevey, the well-known man-about-town, found: 'The quickest motion is to me frightful; it is really flying and it is impossible to divest yourself of the notion of instant death to all upon the least accident happening. It gave me a headache which has not left me yet.' But he admitted that he was in a minority. Another Establishment figure, Charles Greville, was more typical. 'The first sensation is a slight degree of nervousness and a feeling of being run away with, but a sense of security soon supervenes ... it entirely renders all other travelling irksome and tedious by comparison.'

The writer William Thackeray was one of those who grasped how railways represented a break with history, and not only in transport terms.

We who have lived before railways belong to another world ... stage coaches, more or less swift, riding horses, pack-horses, highwaymen, knights in armour, Norman invaders, Roman legions, Druids, Ancient Britons painted blue ... we who lived before railways ... are like Father Noah and his family out of the Ark. ... There will be but ten pre-railroaders left: then three – then two – then one – then O!

This feeling of deep and inevitable change was not new, but had previously been confined to political rather than technical revolutions.

It was not a purely British sentiment. Looking back over a long life Charles Francis Adams pinpointed 1835, the year his native city of Boston was linked to its immediate hinterland by three railroad lines, as 'an historical dividing line. The world we now live in came into existence then; and, humanly speaking, it is, in almost every essential respect, a different world from that lived in by the preceding six generations.'

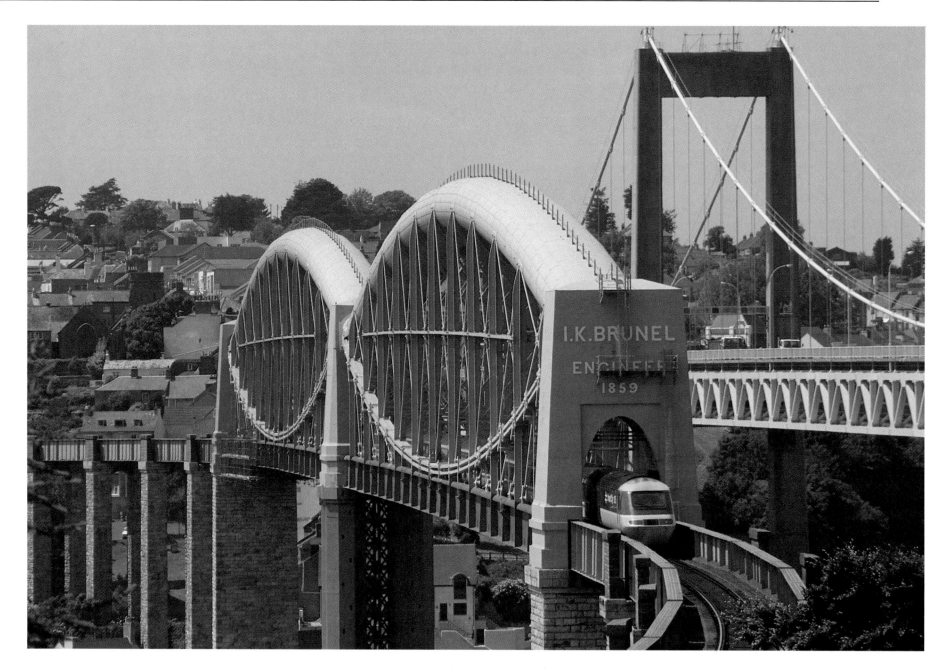

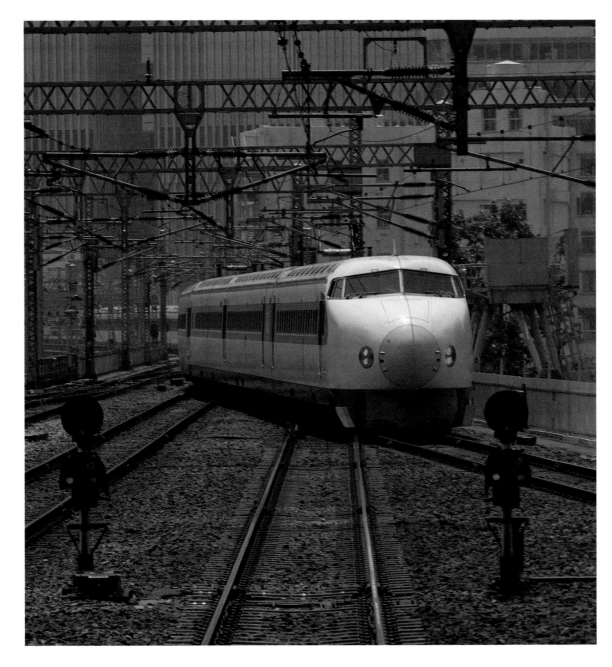

Left *Brunel's last masterpiece, the Saltash Bridge which provided Cornwall with its crucial link to the outside world: still used by the world's fastest diesel trains, the HS125s.*

Right *The magic of modern railways. A Shinkansen (Bullet Train) weaving its way into Tokyo station.*

Practical people, like the novelist R. S. Surtees, rejoiced in the new form of travel. They remembered how 'to be perched for twenty hours, exposed to all weathers, on the outside of a coach, trying in vain to find a soft seat ... was a miserable undertaking.' It was also extremely rough, rougher even than the early trains, with their primitive suspensions (based on those used in horse-drawn carriages) riding on light, carelessly laid rails. Fanny Kemble was exaggerating when she claimed that 'the motion is as smooth as possible. I could either have read or written' – though a generation later Anthony Trollope did manage to write many of his novels on trains.

Nevertheless this entirely new form of transport, which upset every previous notion, soon became embedded in people's everyday lives. It has taken generations for the world to become accustomed to travelling by air, yet it took barely a decade for an earlier generation to take steam in its stride. Within a few years Creevey, like everyone else, was treating a railway journey as a matter of course.

Even the loud and much-publicized opposition to the railways by Britain's landowners turned out to be a matter of money. Their fears that the trains would disturb their hunting and shooting were soon relieved when they were systematically overpaid for every right of way, every piece of land required. It took only a decade to pay them off, a period of time adequate for the railways to render completely irrelevant a recent and itself important and novel form of transport – the stage-coaches travelling on the hard macadamized roads constructed only a few decades earlier. Indeed the railways despatched the stage-coach even more quickly than the jet airliner saw off the propeller-driven aircraft, which, like the stage-coach, had reached its peak of perfection at the very moment it was replaced. The canal systems, first of Britain, and then of the United States and continental Europe, struggled for somewhat longer, but within twenty years they too had lost much of their traffic.

For the railway revolution was both speedy and universal. Twenty years after the first proper passenger service had been inaugurated every major town in Britain had been linked by the iron road, and within another twenty years the same applied to every important town in Western Europe as well – a pace of development far faster than that of the railways' later rivals, the aeroplane and the motorcar.

The railways' first effect was on speed. For the first time in history, men could travel faster than a horse. As Sydney Smith, wittiest and most perceptive of clergymen, noted: 'Before this invention man, richly endowed with many gifts of mind and body, was deficient in locomotive powers … I can now run much faster than a fox or a hare and beat a carrier pigeon or an eagle for a hundred miles.'

For her part Fanny Kemble, who travelled at up to 35 mph (55 kph), claimed that they were travelling faster than any bird 'for they tried the experiment with a snipe'. The effects were both immediate and delayed. Time and again one can discover changes which took place a generation or more after the railways were first built – just as the full effects of computers on people's daily lives had to wait forty years after the invention itself. By themselves the railways were a dynamic force. When combined with other innovations, like the steamship or the Wheatstone telegraph, they were all-conquering.

The railways liberated the human imagination and enlarged man's confidence in dealing with nature. The way that they were built throughout the world, overcoming every obstacle, tunnelling under the Alps, linking oceans through lines thousands of kilometres long, climbing up to 4600 m (15,000 ft) in the Andes – above the level of Mont Blanc – provided a firm nineteenth-century foundation for the assumption equally typical of the present century, that man has the capacity to carry through any scheme he pleases, to defy and conquer nature in all its forms.

1 *The Ideas of Steam*

One of the railway's most crucial attributes, perhaps its most important, was that it was almost universal. Within a few decades it had penetrated into the most peaceful nook. Typically, Nathaniel Hawthorne, sitting in the tranquil woods of Massachusetts, reflected how 'the whistle of the locomotive ... brings the noisy world into the midst of our slumbrous peace.' It was thus far more difficult to escape from the bustle of the urban, increasingly industrialized world. As a result rural tranquillity was the more precious because it could no longer be taken for granted, it had to be fought for against alien intrusions. So it was not surprising that the

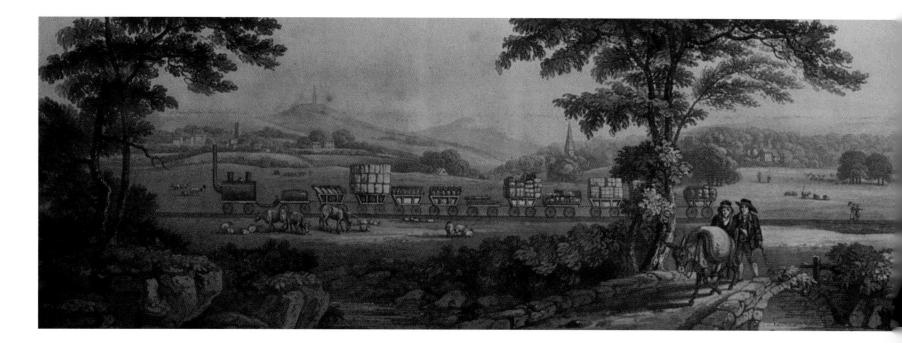

idea of the Nimby (Not In My Back Yard) was created by William Wordsworth in his fight against the intrusion of the railways in the Lake District in the 1840s, nor that half a century later the National Trust was founded as a reaction against a later incursion into that same haven of rural peace.

If the railways were an alien intrusion into nature, then travel by them was logically perceived as alienating the traveller from the natural reality he or she experienced by horse or horse-drawn coach. Ironically, people now say, rightly, that 'you see far more of the country if you travel by train' than by later and even more alienating forms of travel like the car, or, more especially, the aeroplane.

But the initial alienation of travelling by train was felt keenly by a whole generation of intellectuals in France as well as in Britain. Their reaction was summed up by John Ruskin, who wrote, 'All travel becomes dull in exact proportion to its rapidity. Going by railroad I do not consider travelling at all; it is merely "being sent" to a place and not very different from being a parcel.'

(Ruskin's use of 'railroad' is interesting: like many others of his generation he used

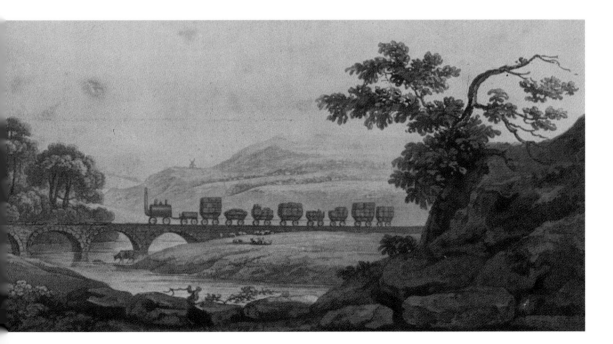

The artist (probably employed by the railway company) ensured that the locomotives on the line from London to Dover appear picturesque – like mobile beer barrels – rather than threatening.

the original word, which remained in use in the United States. In Britain it was soon supplanted by the term 'railway', originally used in publicity material issued by railway promoters anxious to emphasize the private and exclusive nature of their line, as against the word 'road' which implied that the line would be free for use by all comers.)

Ruskin was by no means alone in complaining that the traveller was dehumanized and treated like a parcel. People used to being treated as individuals entitled to special treatment (especially the upper classes) were naturally upset at being lumped together, compartmentalized both figuratively, as merely one amongst a general body of persons, and literally, travelling in compartments like anyone else. For travelling by rail involved what could seem like a Faustian pact with the devil of steam: in return for freedom from the limits in terms of speed and time previously imposed by Nature, rail travellers had to accept all manner of restrictions: to travel only when the train (or rather its operators) chose, to sit where they were put, with other people whom they did not necessarily know, to apply for tickets and to obey a wide variety of laws, by-laws and restrictions before, during and after the journey.

Railways brought with them, in their train as it were, many standardized elements requiring precision and discipline. You queued for a ticket, you obeyed the guard or the porter when he told you to embark and to disembark. And these men were not independent, they were merely servants of an implacable mechanical machine, bigger than them, composed not only of the locomotives and the trains themselves but also of an organized hierarchy.

For railways inevitably industrialized travel, and in doing so standardized it. They introduced the notion of an industrially regulated society throughout the world, where previously it had been confined to a small number of urban industrial centres, mostly in northern England. But their most obvious effect was the standardization of time. No longer could peasants and their masters live by the rhythm of the sun. If railways were to provide a regular service they had, necessarily, to conform to some form of schedule, and that meant bringing order into the chaos that was time before railways, in which every town prided itself on keeping its own time, a few minutes different from a neighbour a few miles away. The railways' imposition of this important piece of standardization had to wait twenty years or so for another invention, the Wheatstone telegraph, whose wires marched parallel to the railway tracks the world over and which enabled exact times to be transmitted instantly to the most distant station.

The adoption of standard time was less dramatic in such relatively small countries as Britain or France than it was in the United States, where it was so important that the convention which first met to consider the question in 1872 was the forerunner of the industry's present trade body, the Association of American Railroads. In October 1883 the AAR adopted what they called the General Time Convention, dividing the continent into four broad zones, and the new divisions were introduced a mere five weeks later. It took the United States Congress a further twenty-five years to legalize the process, for in imposing their own ideas the railroads had acted as independent authorities, not relying on government decisions.

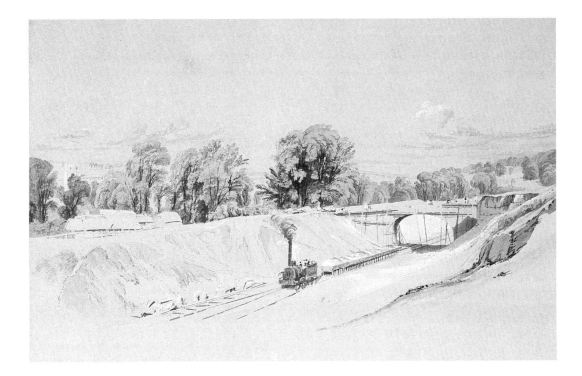

One of Thomas Bourne's most evocative scenes, of the Berkhamsted cutting, one of the many on the line from London to Birmingham.

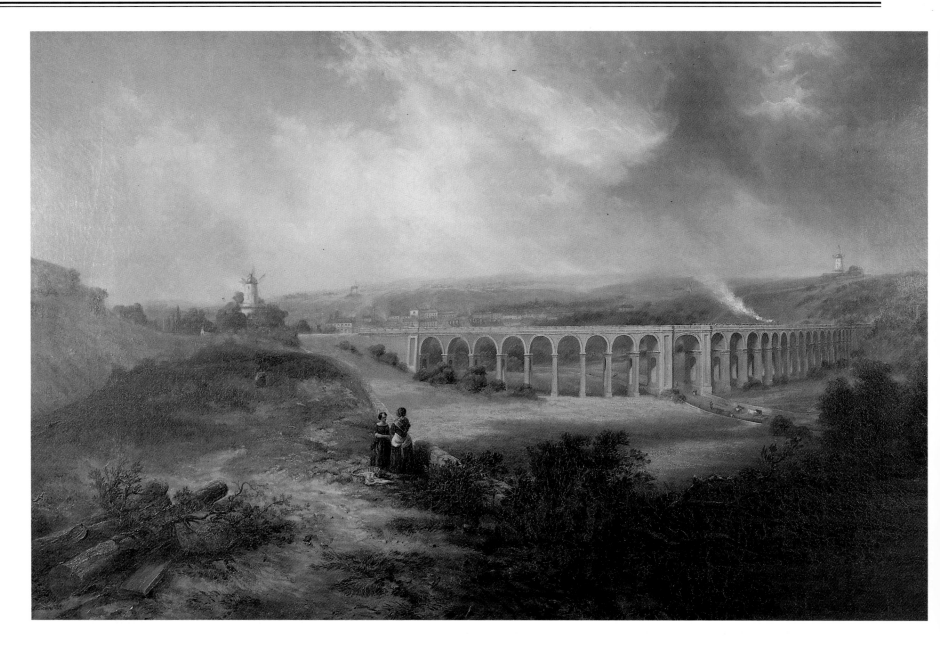

John Wilson Carmichael's delightful view of the London Road Viaduct on another pioneering line, from London to Brighton.

Not surprisingly, almost before any of them had actually been built, railways were perceived as the spirit, the 'genius' of the emerging age – the age of steam. Henry Booth, the treasurer of the Liverpool & Manchester Railway, set the tone in 1830 for many subsequent expressions of the feeling.

> The locomotive engine and railway were reserved for the present day. From west to east, and from north to south, the mechanical principle, the philosophy of the nineteenth century, will spread and extend itself. The world has received a new impulse. The genius of the age, like a mighty river of a new world, flows onward, full, rapid and irresistible.

If only today's finance directors could write like that!

The railways speedily upset that most fundamental of perceptions: the relation between time, speed and distance. Again it was Henry Booth who best articulated the new order:

> Perhaps the most striking result produced by the completion of the railway is the sudden and marvellous change which has been effected in our ideas of time and space. Notions which we have received from our ancestors, and verified by our own experience, are overthrown in a day . . . our notions of expedition, though at first having reference to locomotion, will influence . . . more or less, the whole tenor and business of life.

Railways did indeed represent the spirit of the age, did indeed effect many seemingly miraculous transformations. But neither they, nor any subsequent invention, could change the ingrained essence of a society. They did indeed standardize, centralize, but not nearly as dramatically as their supporters had hoped. For they were usually not in themselves revolutionary forces. In most instances they simply enabled revolutions brought by other causes to spread more easily and completely. One can see in this delusion of the all-devouring, all-powerful mechanical force the precursor of the arrogance of the prophecies attached to a series of other scientific innovations over the years, from television to the computer. The changes they create are manifold and undeniable, but – much to the chagrin of determinists – they leave untouched many of the fundamental attributes which make us human. Indeed they often turn out either to be neutral, or to enable the human spirit – in all its aspects, for good or ill – to express itself more fully.

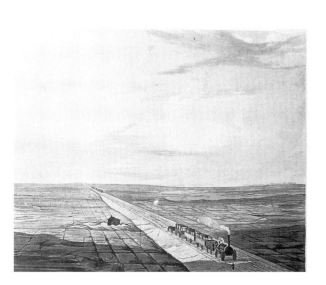

T. J. Bury's print exaggerates the desolation of Chat Moss. Laying tracks across the marsh between Liverpool and Manchester was a triumph for George Stephenson.

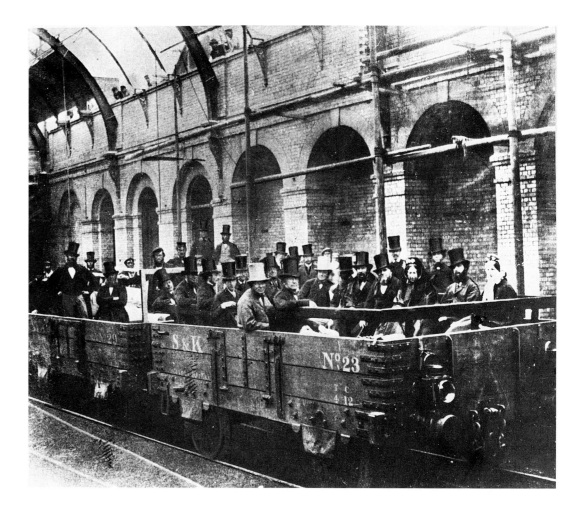

William Gladstone (between the men in tall white hats) in 1862 on the first trial run of the world's first underground railway, from Paddington Station to Moorgate in the City of London.

For instance, the relationships between the state and the railways reflected the basic notions which already prevailed in the countries concerned. Typically, the Anglo-Saxons responded very differently from their counterparts in continental Europe. Alone in Europe Britain allowed the market to rule. Parliament intervened only to provide the legal rights required to acquire charters and permission for new lines, and, belatedly and inadequately, to supervise the railway companies. For the railway lobby was powerful – powerful enough to ensure that one over-conscientious Inspector-General of Railways was dismissed. In Jack Simmons' words, 'he had shown himself shrewd, untiring and incorruptible. No wonder the railway chairmen and managers disliked him.'

Surprisingly, the independence of the railway companies in both Britain and the United States was little affected by the fact that they depended on the government, in Britain because every new line required a separate Act of Parliament and in the United States because so many of them depended heavily on the federal government for land grants to finance their construction. But both countries accepted the price of capitalist competition: massive and wasteful duplication, particularly in the United States where a dozen or more competing routes ran between major cities like New York and Chicago.

Virtually everywhere else in the world the prevailing national culture was more corporate, less market-oriented. As railways were deemed of overriding national import-ance, they were treated from the start as national, rather than private organizations; the state would often provide concessions to the promoters for a fixed period of years, after which the lines would revert to national ownership.

Typically, the French laid only a few minor lines until they had determined the principles on which their national network should be built – with the inevitable result that they centred on Paris, providing inadequate links between many of the most important provincial towns. But the national framework did ensure that the lines were not expensively duplicated, and that they did provide major centres with efficient links with the capital. Moreover when, as usually happened, the early promoters ran out of money, the state stepped in to provide a framework to protect them.

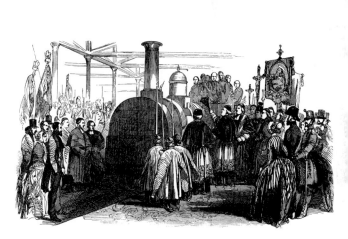

The Catholic Church never opposed railways. Inevitably the bishop blessed the line from Rouen to Le Havre in 1847.

The differences in national attitudes also reflected very different ideas of the relation-ship between individuals and large organizations (whether privately or publicly-owned). In Britain the railways were presumed to be a service provided for the traveller, while elsewhere in Europe they were provided, if not by an all-powerful state, by a company which took on a pseudo-social mantle and was thus felt to be entitled to obedience.

The result was a marked contrast between the relative freedom assumed by Anglo-Saxons, especially at stations, and the more orderly, disciplined ways of the other nations, even supposedly anarchic Latin races like the French and the Italians. While waiting for their train the British and the Americans could wander about the platform with their baggage. In France travellers had to surrender their baggage and wait in their appointed waiting room until they were liberated – like airline passengers today, by order of classes.

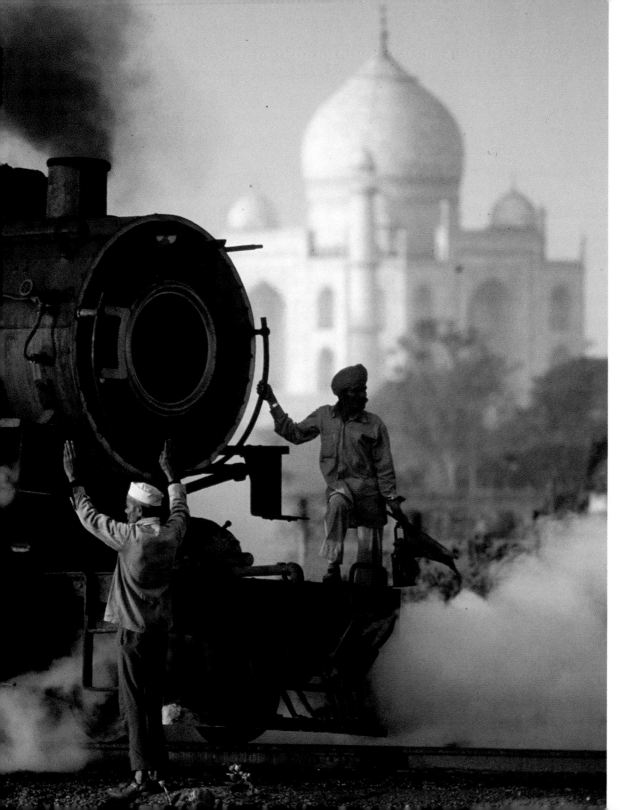

The stuff of mystic reflections about dreams and reality: the contrast between the timeless Taj Mahal and the down-to-earth railways.

*F*iguratively as well as literally, railways were thought to be a uniquely effective means of binding together the many new countries which emerged during their Golden Age, between 1830 and the end of the nineteenth century. The pattern was set by Belgium which wrested its independence from the Dutch in 1830. From the start the Belgians defined their country through their plan for a national rail network, designed not only to bind the country together but also to free the new country from Dutch domination by providing an alternative means of transport if the Dutch blocked the waterways between Antwerp and the North Sea.

As a result Belgium became a model 'railway country' industrially as well as politically: its industrial importance in the nineteenth century, when Belgian names like Belpaire and Walschaerts were world-famous, and its decline in the twentieth, were both due to this reliance. But, socially, the railways remained a symbol of the Belgium-that-never-was. However carefully planned the network, it has never had any real influence in diminishing the tribal allegiances felt by the French-speaking Walloons in the south and the Flemish-speaking people in the north which remain as strong today as they were a century and a half ago.

Thirty years after the Belgians had attempted their exercise in unification through railways, the Italians made the same experiment, with hardly more success. Count Cavour, the architect of Italian unity, was a railway fanatic – at one point he even drew up the timetables for the country's embryonic railway system. And in the decades after Italian unification in 1860 the railways developed as a conscious unifying force. Cavour, like his Italian successors and their equivalent elsewhere in the world, was not too fussy about actual ownership. He recognized that private capital was essential, provided only – a difficult point to establish with the promoters – that it did not reduce the government's long-term control over the tracks. Although the development of a network in a mountainous country demonstrated to the full the Italian genius for civil engineering it did not stop Italy remaining a profoundly regionalized country – as witness the rise of the Lombard League in the past few years.

The most obvious example of a country conceived by the railway is Canada. It was, and remains, true that 'without a railroad there is no Canada', and indeed three provinces, including far-off British Columbia, joined the Federation only after they had been guaranteed a rail link to the rest of the country. Moreover the Canadians used the development of their railway system not only to assert their national identity but also to ensure that they were not overly dominated by their giant southern neighbour. Time and again they rejected shorter, cheaper, and more economically viable routes across the country because they were not purely Canadian but passed through the northern United States. Later, the Canadians' obsession with railways as a unifying force was to cost them dear when they decided that the (purely Canadian) Canadian Pacific Railway, the very model of a transcontinental railway, efficient, honestly built, economically constructive, was inadequate, as well as being a monopoly. So vast sums were poured into the development of a northern alternative, the Canadian National Railway, the perfect example of a railway which helped develop previously barren lands but was never going to be commercially viable.

By no coincidence, Belgium, Italy and Canada, the three countries which used railways most consciously to assert what their creators must have known was a largely artificial national identity, are still – indeed increasingly – fissiparous, their unity increasingly threatened by centrifugal forces threatening to break them apart.

The symbolic importance of railways was not confined to Europe. In Latin America they were treated as a symbol of liberation from foreign interference, as a matter of prestige (like nationally-owned airlines since 1945) and of peace between potential rivals. When the Trans-Andean line between Chile and Argentina was finally opened in 1913 a bronze statue of Christ was erected on the summit of the Cumbre, the fearsome mountain separating the two countries. The inscription told all: 'Sooner shall these mountains crumble into dust than the people of Argentina and Chile break the peace which they have sworn to maintain at the feet of Christ the redeemer.' And in his comprehensive survey *Railways of the World*, published a year earlier, Ernest Protheroe described the occasion as 'one of the great victories of peace, that will bind the nations closer in social and commercial progress, thus rendering their oath easier to keep'.

Although railways could not forge an artificial unity amongst a diverse group of people who happened to be living in a defined geographical entity, they could be powerful symbols of progress and unity, for railways could have a considerable effect if they were working with the national grain. In France it was the development of the 'Freycinet lines', named after the politician who raised the finance for a massive network of minor rural lines in the 1870s, which finally united the whole of France, ensuring (surprisingly for the first time) that almost all Frenchmen spoke the same language, and not a series of dialects.

Railways played an enormous part in the unification of Germany. Otto von Bismarck, the creator of united Germany, saw that railways were far too important to be left either to the market or to the individual states he brought together, and he fought long, hard and successfully to provide the country with a unified network under national control.

But perhaps the best European example of the role railways could play in defining a country's politics came in Switzerland. The country's first railways were developed by outsiders, principally French and German industrialists and bankers, and the result, as in so many other less developed countries, was furious nationalist agitation against the foreigners' actual and supposed misdeeds. The resulting vote at the end of the nineteenth century which brought Switzerland's railways under state control was a watershed in increasing the role of the federal government in the nation's affairs.

Japan provides an even better illustration of the way a country redefined itself through its progress in grappling with the problems of building and operating railways. The Japanese started from scratch: in 1853, when Commander Perry arrived on his first voyage, the country had never seen a wheeled vehicle, and there was no tradition of industrial discipline. Unbelievable as it may now seem, a phrasebook published as late as 1898 contained the following exchange: 'Why can't you start punctually?' To which the answer ran: 'Unpunctuality is a Japanese habit and there is no help for it.'

But progress was swift. On his second visit in 1854 Commander Perry brought with him a quarter-size miniature locomotive and train, complete with track, as a present for the Emperor. And that same year a Dutch book containing information about steam engines was translated into Japanese. Fourteen years later one of the first steps of the new Meiji government in its determination to modernize the country was to build a railway between Tokyo and Yokohama.

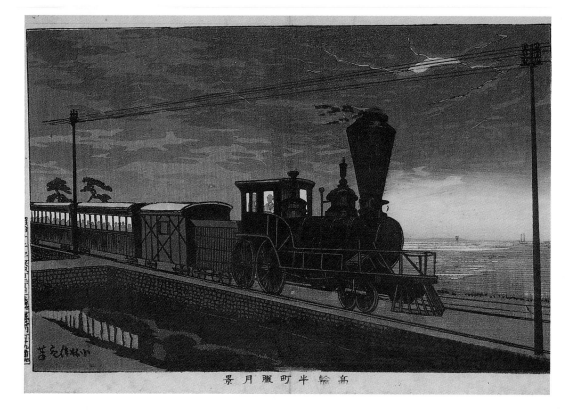

景月朧町半輪高

The western dream visualized by the Japanese artist Kiyochika. Note the charming, almost Impressionistic, inaccuracy of the locomotive's wheels.

The backwardness of the Japanese and the speed of their progress were both extraordinary to Western eyes. The first rickshaw ran in 1870, the first steam locomotive two years later – and the first electric tramway as early as 1895, by which time Japan had virtually caught up with the West. Twelve years earlier the British engineer B. R. F Wright paid a notable tribute after his Japanese pupils had built a turbine and compressor: 'The whole work has been made and erected by, and is now in entire charge of men who eleven years ago had not seen a railway or machinery for making them.' For the Japanese, typically, relied on foreign expertise and foreign capital for the shortest possible time: within a decade they had redeemed the only loan they had raised, which was used to finance their first line, a degree of financial self-reliance unique amongst developing countries.

All the hopes attached to the development of railways and their importance to a new country were most fully expressed in the United States. The Americans had started work

Opposite Go West Young Man. *As Currier & Ives visualized the march of the rails towards an ever-changing horizon.*

30

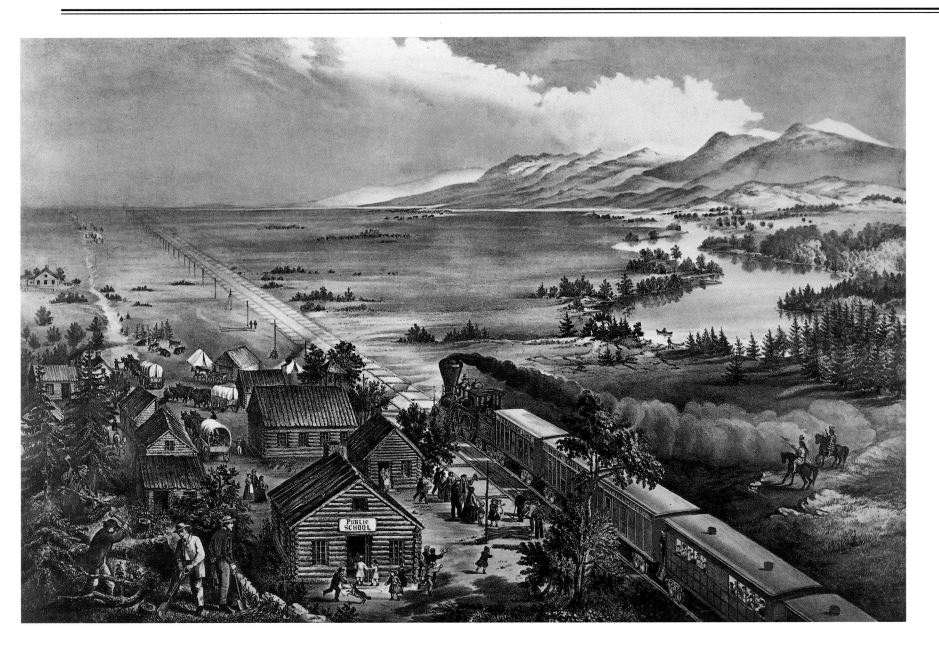

on railways early, and their future importance was properly symbolized when Charles Carroll, the last surviving signatory of the Declaration of Independence, dug the first spadeful of earth for the first line (from Baltimore inland into Ohio), appropriately enough on Independence Day in 1828.

From the very start the railway was seen as the fullest expression of the American dream, of the nation's vigour, of the compatibility of public good and private enterprise. They prided themselves on being a 'locomotive' people. Mrs Houstoun, a British visitor of the 1850s, wrote:

> I really thought there must be some natural affinity between Yankee 'keep-moving' nature and a locomotive engine ... Whatever the cause it is certain that the humans seem to treat the 'ingine', as they call it, more like a familiar friend than as the dangerous and desperate thing it really is.

In 1847 D. Kimball Minor, the editor of the *American Railroad Journal*, described the railroad thus: 'Greater than any, we may say all other means – of perpetuating our glorious union. It will prove literally ... as bands of iron binding us together, a family of states – thus ensuring our greatness and permanence as a nation.'

The greatness, the permanence and the unity were most strikingly shown in the first transcontinental railroad. For the railways' importance was far more than symbolic. As the Americans were only too acutely aware, theirs was not a naturally united continent. Only a railway system could provide a framework for defining as well as uniting the continent. Not surprisingly every major city, none more obviously than Washington, boasted a Union Station. Abraham Lincoln totally understood the point. He attached enormous importance to the Pacific Railroad Act of 1862 which led within seven short years to the completion of the Transcontinental Railroad.

The Act was passed in the middle of a Civil War which comprehensively rubbed in the country's natural disunity. For behind the booster language was the fact that in their first century of existence the supposedly 'united' states were haunted by a fear of disintegration. In a survey of the literature promoting railways called *Railroads and the Character of America*, James A. Ward observed that many of them 'radiate an almost desperate energy, an intimation that railways might be the last hope for holding the political experiment together.' As Albro Martin wrote in *Railroads Triumphant*:

> It had a dramatically different purpose from any of the railroad ventures up to that time. It was undertaken by the people as a national enterprise. [The two railway companies involved] ... were authorized by Congress as Civil War measures, intended to bind the Pacific coast tier of states ... more closely to the Union. It had been impossible for most people to imagine an American republic occupying the entire continent from ocean to ocean before the coming of the railroad.

But the Transcontinental also marked a profound shift towards private enterprise. The National Road, an earlier attempt to construct a road to the mid-west, had been entirely in the public sector. By contrast, as Seymour Dunbar pointed out in *A History of Travel in America Vol I* in 1937, the Transcontinental 'was built by a less direct exercise of national authority, through corporate instrumentalities created by the nation for the purpose, and to which the government delegated powers which it had in the previous instance used in its own person.'

But the railroads were also psychologically crucial. According to Ward:

> The new form of transport could unite discordant images. Railways could at the same time serve individual betterment and the public good. By spending public monies freely, the nation could promote sturdier individualism. Ideas would travel as far and as fast as merchandise.

The feeling reached a climax on 10 May 1869 when the United States was finally linked at Promontory Point, Utah, a moment when the whole continent held its breath, when elaborate arrangements were made to telegraph the precise moment at which the rails were joined by the symbolic Golden Spike, a moment celebrated throughout the continent. Dunbar was not exaggerating when he wrote:

> If those of future times should seek for a day on which the country at last became a nation ... it may be that they will not select the verdict of some political campaign or battle-field but choose, instead, the hour when two engines – one from the East and the other from the West – met at Promontory.

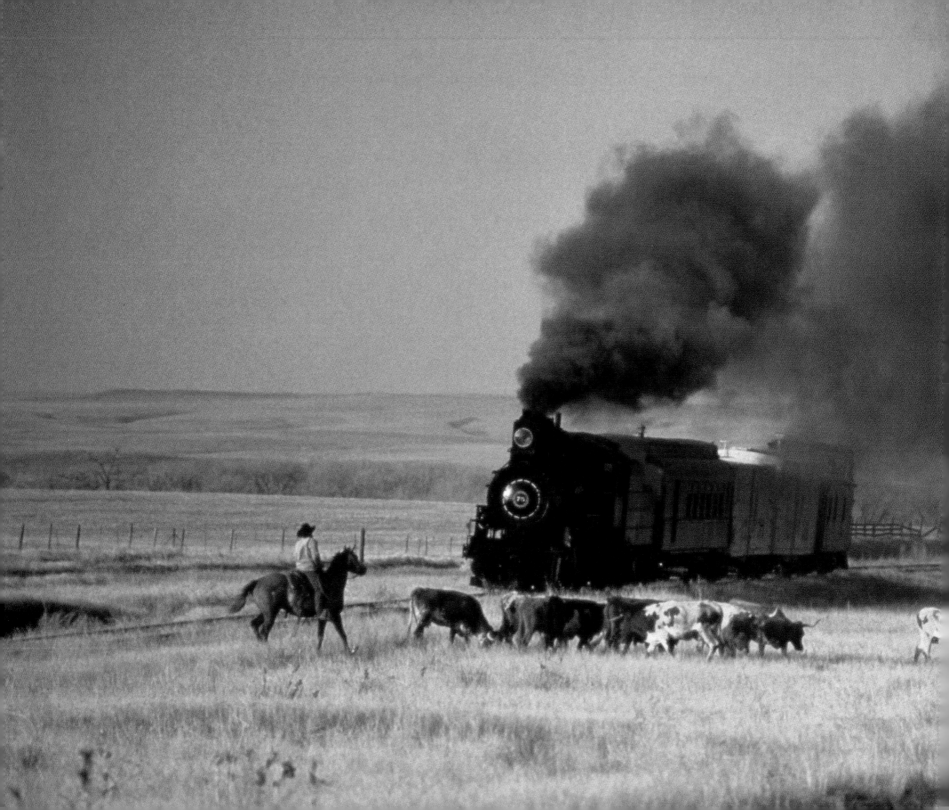

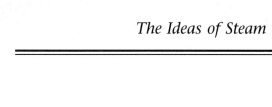

The more-or-less-real West – remember the song from Oklahoma!*: 'The corn is as high as an elephant's eye.'*

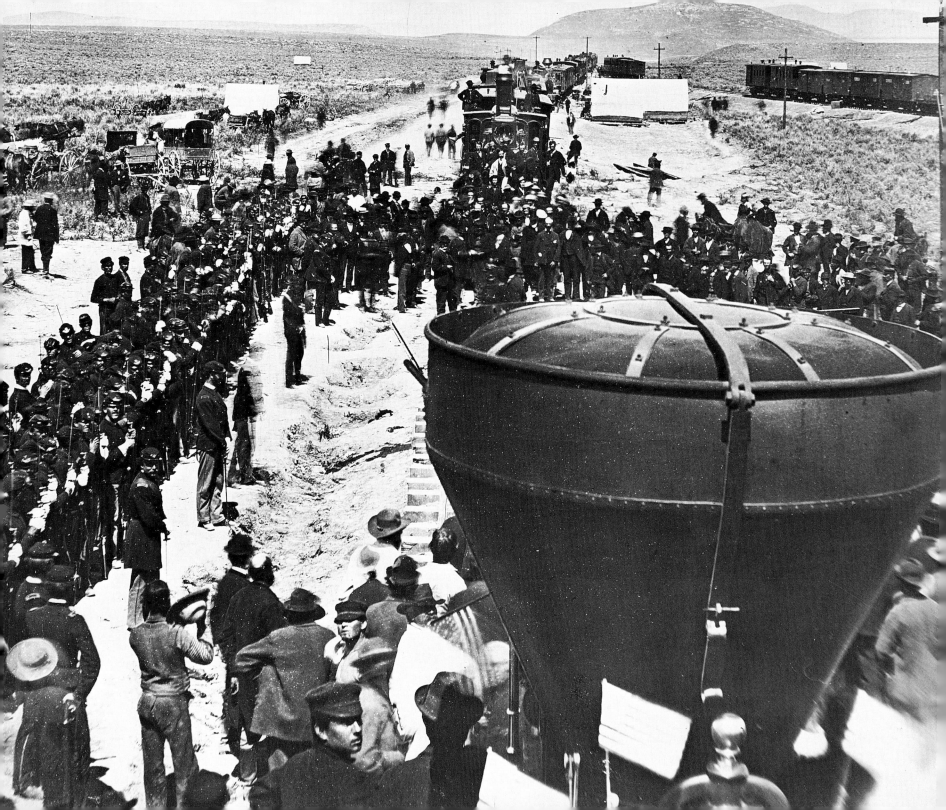

Not surprisingly railroads entered into the language more fully than any subsequent mechanical invention. As early as the 1850s it was so impregnated with railway lore that the trail by which negroes were smuggled north and away from their slavemasters was known as the 'underground railroad', and not just because freight cars were often used as means of transport. Slaves were cared for at 'stations', the owners were known as 'agents', the men who escorted the slaves from one station to another as 'conductors', while the slaves themselves were known as 'passengers'.

Half a century later the 'Railroad man's prayer' in *The Railroad Man's Magazine* managed to include a dozen such terms:

> Now that I have flagged Thee, lift up my feet from the road of life and plant them safely on the deck of the train of salvation. Let me use the safety lamp of prudence, make all couplings with the link of love, let my hand-lamp be my Bible, and keep all switches closed that lead off the main line into the sidings with blind ends. Have every semaphore white along the line of hope, that I may make the run of life without stopping. Give me the Ten Commandments as a working card, and when I have finished the run on schedule time and pulled into the terminal, may Thou, superintendent of the universe, say: 'well done, good and faithful servant, come into the general office to sign the pay-roll and receive your check for happiness.'

The folklore of railways remained powerful. Until the arrival of the gramophone record in the early twentieth century many hit songs concerned railway disasters involving daring anti-heroes like Casey Jones. Later, jazz travelled along the railway line from New Orleans to Kansas City, and, above all, to Chicago. As Paul Theroux wrote in *The Old Patagonian Express*:

Left *The Birth of the Nation. After the tracks of the first railway across the newly-United States had been joined by the legendary Golden Spike at Promontory Point, Utah.*

Below *Jazz travelled north, by train from New Orleans – though not usually in such picturesque trains.*

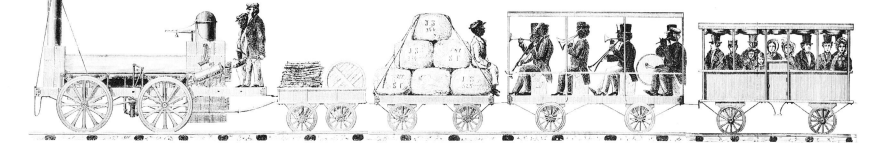

Opposite *The Durango & Silverton Railway in Colorado once served the local mines but is now one of the United States' prime tourist attractions.*

... half of jazz is railway music, and the motion and noise of the train itself has the rhythm of jazz. This is not surprising: the Jazz age was also the railway age. Musicians travelled by train or not at all and the pumping tempi and the clickety clack and the lonesome whistle crept into the songs.

It was a stroke of genius to recreate the song from Bizet in *Carmen Jones*: 'Hear the train along the track, clickety clack, clickety clack, it only takes a half a day to be a thousand miles away' – significantly 'on the Chicago train'.

The repertoire of rail-connected songs sank deeply into the American subconscious. When Elizabeth Cotten sang *Freight train run so fast* during Senate hearings on the Folklore Preservation Act, the whole audience, including the senators, joined in the singing without prompting. They knew not only the words, but also the sub-text.

Long after the actual tracks have been abandoned by all but a handful of passengers American politicians remain aware of the powerful symbolism attached to the railways. To take one obvious example: Presidential candidates have been conducting their campaigns from the back of railway trains criss-crossing the continent for a century or more. In the 1992 Presidential election, President Bush used the cabooses of trains from which to address the electors. In doing so he was consciously reverting to the populist style of campaigning last seen in 1948 when Harry Truman, Bush's model, used the same platform on his 'Give 'em hell' tour which bought him such unexpected success. Truman's method of transport was a natural one for his day and age. Forty-four years later Bill Clinton, the successful Democratic challenger, was being more natural in campaigning by bus, using the system of interstate highways which had in the meantime almost completely replaced the railroads for passenger transport.

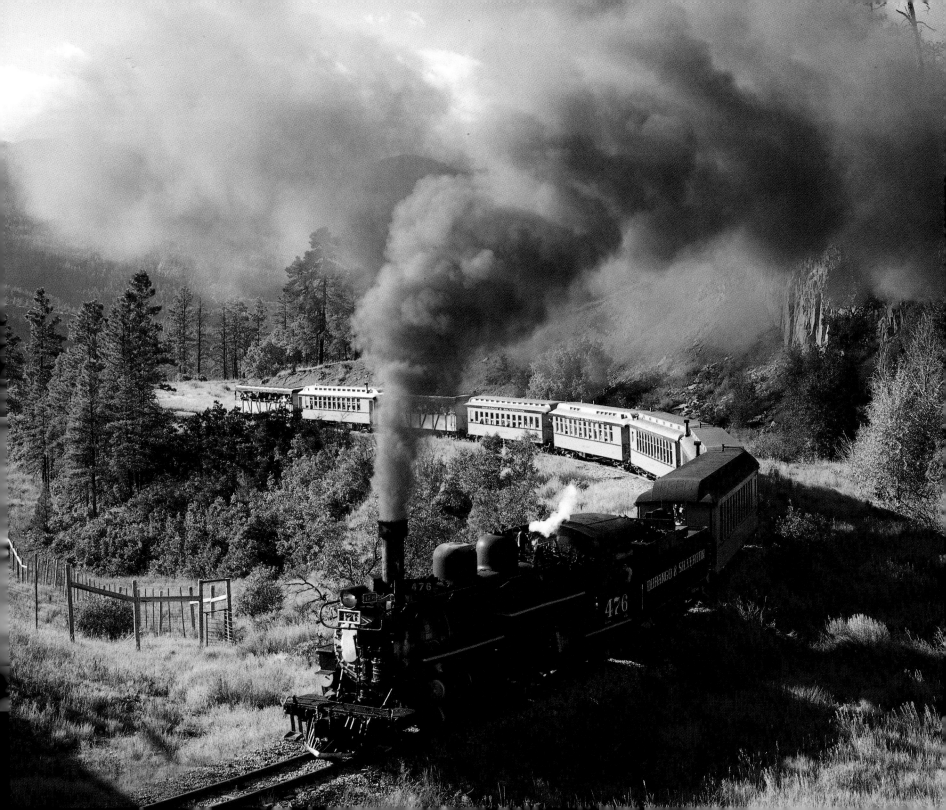

2 Men of Steam

The railways created new breeds of men: engineers – usually unsung – contractors, the promoters and bankers behind them, and the managers who ran the railway systems. All were extraordinary themselves. All left legacies. These could be physical, the lines and the buildings associated with them; or, in the case of the promoters and the managers, systems which, for good or ill, we recognize as the prototypes of today's financial markets and corporate world.

Railways were not built by machines, but by men, millions of them. Only in the late nineteenth century, at the end of the railways' heroic age, did machines driven by steam reinforce the picks and shovels wielded by the navvies whose blood and sweat had already been responsible for thousands of miles of lines.

But the labourers were not the first characters on the railway scene. In the beginning, as the novelist George Eliot remembered forty years later, were those mysterious beings, the surveyors and the engineers who commanded them.

> One or two strange faces appeared in the town [Watford, then a peaceful Hertfordshire community] and men in leathern leggings, dragging a long chain, and attended by one or two country labourers armed with bill-hooks, were remarked as trespassing in the most unwarrantable manner over pasture land, standing crops, copse and cover; actually cutting gaps in the hedges, through which they climbed and dragged the land-chain. Then would follow another intruder, bearing a telescope set on three legs, which he erected with the most perfect coolness wherever he thought fit.

The navvies who followed close on the heels of the surveyors were a community apart. The name and the reality were created by the construction of Britain's canal system at the end of the eighteenth century. But the railways in Britain – let alone the rest of

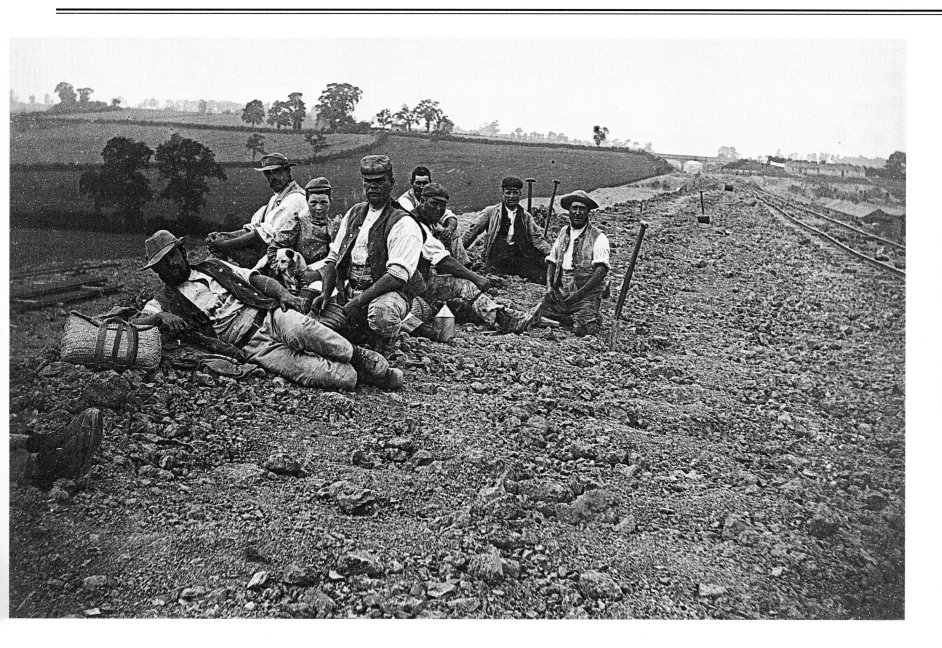

The last of the real navvies, captured by S. W. A. Newton on the Great Central from Marylebone to Sheffield at the end of the nineteenth century.

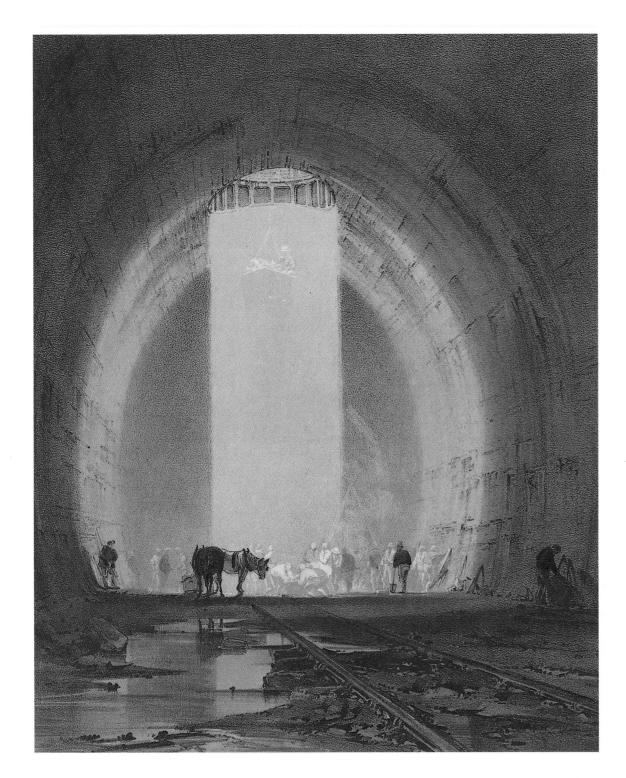

The working shaft of the Kilsby Tunnel on the London to Birmingham Railway as seen by Thomas Bourne – the most dramatic image depicting the early days of railway construction.

the world – required far more 'navigators'. They came from the oppressed of the earth: from any country, most obviously Ireland, China and, later, India, which was poor, grossly overpopulated, their people used to hard lives engaged in back-breaking manual labour. Only in Russia were massive railway systems built with native labour, in this case by thousands of serfs. After the Revolution they were replaced by political prisoners when Stalin extended the Russian railway system hundreds of miles to the Arctic coal mines.

They were all lumped together under the name of navvies, but they were not merely diggers, since the work of railway construction required masons, bridge-builders, shot-firers, lumberjacks and men with the specialist skills required to lay the actual tracks. In the words of Samuel Smiles in his *Lives of the Engineers*: 'Their expertness in all sorts of earthwork, in embanking, boring and well-sinking – their practical knowledge of the nature of soils and rocks, the tenacity of clays, and the porosity of certain stratifications – were very great.'

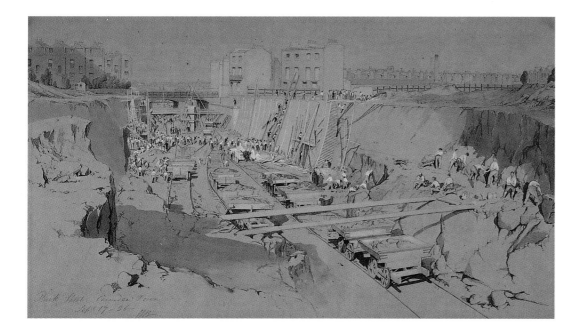

Building a wall so solid it still retains the embankment at Camden Town on the London to Birmingham Railway.

The Irish, who dominated the heroic age of railway-building throughout the world, had already proved themselves as doughty diggers before the great famine of 1845–46, provided their employers with a mass of recruits anxious to escape their impoverished homeland at all costs. At the same time China was visited by more than its usual share of flood, famine and civil wars, which triggered off an exodus to the West Coast of the United States. Here railway builders were desperate for labour following the California Gold Rush in 1849 – although the railways built from the East through the Prairies in the late 1860s could rely on the army of ex-soldiers left unemployed after the end of the Civil War.

A 'hotel train' for the engineers and supervisors building the Union Pacific across Nevada in 1864 – the Chinese coolies had to make do with the tents.

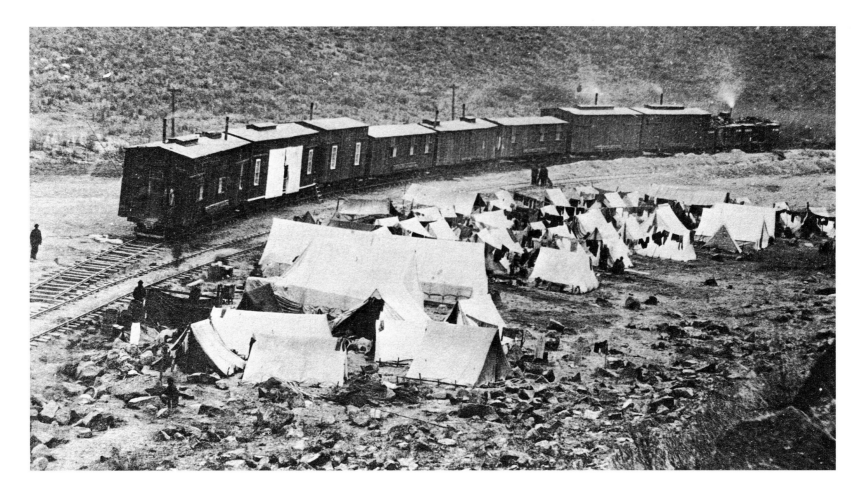

To some, none more so than Samuel Smiles, these men were romantic figures. He describes how the typical navvy:

> ... wandered about from one public work to another – apparently belonging to no country and having no home. He usually wore a white felt hat with the brim turned up, a velveteen or jean square-tailed coat, a scarlet plush waistcoat with little black spots, and a bright-coloured kerchief round his herculean neck, when, as often happened, it was not left entirely bare ... their powers of endurance were extraordinary ... in times of emergency they would work for twelve and even sixteen hours, with only short intervals for meals.

Smiles reckoned that in building the line from London to Birmingham they shifted more rock, earth and stones in five years than had been required for the pyramids at Giza – which had taken four times as long. But then heroic efforts were commonplace on every major railway project. In his book on the Canadian National Railway G. R. Stevens records how one gang 'would work right through the hours of daylight, which in summer meant from three in the morning to nine or ten at night' without any breaks, merely gulping meat like a dog. 'Total elapsed time preparing dinner, three minutes. Total elapsed time eating, nothing.'

Inevitably the navvies 'worked hard and played hard'. Their regular pay-night binges became legendary and they were the terror of the peaceful rural countryside through which they passed. They occupied the same place in local folklore as the evacuees from London and other major cities in the Second World War, both untamed reminders to the more genteel country people of the brute reality of urban working-class life. But the navvies, if not the evacuees, could be pretty frightening. Even their great admirer, Samuel Smiles, described their pay nights as a 'saturnalia of riot and disorder, dreaded by the inhabitants of the villages along the line of works.'

For they moved as roving bands, with their own customs, which, in Britain at least, often included rough marriage ceremonies. This was not always the case elsewhere: in East Africa the Indian navvies were apt to have carnal relations with natives of both sexes, a habit which at least one tribe, the Nandi, took sufficiently amiss to take a murderous revenge on their tormentors.

After enduring the horrors of an emigrant train across the United States, Robert Louis

Stevenson observed 'how in these uncouth places pig-tailed Chinese pirates worked side by side with border ruffians and broken men from Europe, talking together in a mixed dialect, mostly oaths, gambling, drinking, quarrelling and murdering like wolves.' For their presence was by no means conducive to good race relations, to say the least. In the United States the two races principally involved, the Irish and the Chinese, were alike only in their capacity for hard work. The Irish relaxed by drinking, hard and often, the Chinese by gambling and taking opium. The Irish took their revenge on their rivals by setting off explosive charges in cuttings to undermine the Chinese, as if the regular work was not dangerous enough.

For the navvies' life was not really romantic: they could be sure that they would be injured, if not crippled, during a working life which rarely lasted more than a couple of decades. If they were building tunnels then the chance of survival was even lower: workers on the St Gotthard rarely lasted more than a few months.

Outside Europe life was even shorter and more dangerous. Before the days of quinine, let alone antibiotics, the death rate in building railways in the tropics was inevitably staggering. In India nearly a third of the 30,000 to 40,000 labourers working on one particular line died in the course of the rainy season of 1859–1860. But the record was set by the Panama railway, where at one point one worker in five was dying every month. The legend has it that there was 'the body of a navvy under every sleeper' of the infamous railway across the Isthmus and the railway's only doctor financed his hospital by selling pickled corpses in barrels wholesale to medical schools the world over.

*I*n charge of the navvies were the engineers. Throughout the world they had in common a great daring, a singular confidence in themselves and an incredible capacity for hard work – which, however, was often not enough to prevent them dying young of sheer overwork, after long months of twenty-hour days, of endless journeys on rough roads in bouncing carriages.

To the British the description of 'railway engineer' applies above all to George Stephenson (and to a lesser extent his son Robert) and Isambard Kingdom Brunel. In fact, by the standards of his successors, George Stephenson was not a great engineer: he

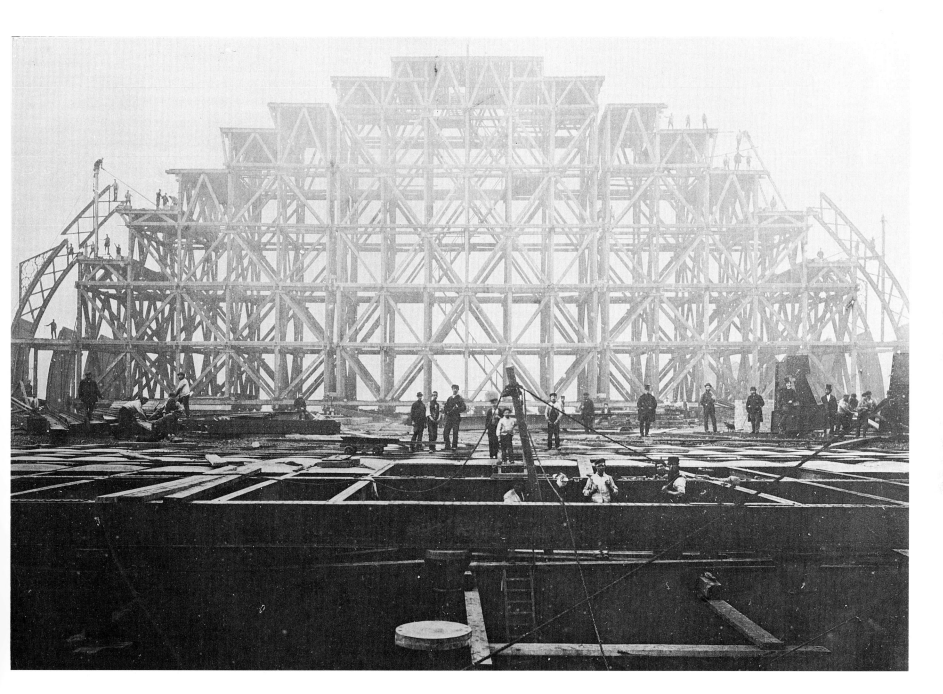

*Building the scaffolding for the engine shed at St Pancras – the steel beams
formed the roof of the cellars for the beer brought from Burton on Trent.*

was a man with an extraordinary fixity of purpose, an iron will, who developed existing ideas and forced them on to an often unwilling public through sheer force of character. By contrast his son Robert was an excellent mechanical engineer who developed his father's locomotives so that they became the models of every steam engine built for a hundred years or more. It was noticeable that when the son emigrated to Latin America for a couple of years to escape his father's overweening influence George made virtually no progress. It was Robert who was responsible for the family's greatest feat of construction, the line from London to Birmingham, even though he was not as great a civil engineer as his immediate successors, like Joseph Locke.

Brunel was the greatest of the three, a man of a vision – and a capacity to realize it – unequalled in the nineteenth century. He dreamed of his railway from London to Bristol as only part of a great chain, from London to Bristol and then on a ship he himself had designed and built – the *Great Western* – to the United States.

His particular genius lay in his capacity to translate so much of his vision into practice. His line from London to Bristol and then on to Exeter showed the world the potential of a railway line: by 1846 trains were running the 200 miles (320 km) from London to Exeter in a mere five hours at an average speed of over 40 mph (65 kph). The station he designed at Paddington in west London is one of the handful which show any real originality of design; and, for all their problems, the steamships he designed were noble visions. But even Brunel was not the all-round Renaissance genius of his dreams. For, from the beginning, railways, the very prototype of modern industry, imposed their own specializations on even their greatest geniuses. He was lucky that his faithful engine superintendent, Daniel Gooch, managed to adapt his master's ideas to reality. The specifications for the locomotives he required were unrealistic, if only because he simply had to be different, as he had been so successfully in imposing a 214 cm (7 ft) gauge for his line to Bristol.

The excessive publicity lavished on the founding trio of engineers has rather concealed the qualities of their successors, mostly to be found outside Britain where the challenges were much more dramatic. The railways in France, and in a number of other European countries, including Spain and the Austro-Hungarian empire, were built by leading graduates from the French engineering schools, the Ecole Polytechnique and the Ecole des Ponts et Chaussées, establishments without any equivalent, then or now, in Britain.

Yet who today has heard of Paulin Talabot, the genius behind the line from Paris to Lyon and Marseilles? Even less well-known is Fulgence Bienvenue who was responsible for the speed with which the Paris Métro was built at the end of the nineteenth century. A typical product of the Ecole Polytechnique, he had lost an arm in a railway accident early in his career. His greatest contribution to engineering science was to devise a system to ensure that the tracks could be built a few metres below street level without disturbing the traffic too badly – shafts were dug at regular intervals and galleries dug outwards from them.

He and his like remain relatively unknown because of the superiority of the French system, by which engineers have always been recognized as natural members of the national managerial hierarchy, and therefore not likely to be chosen as especially heroic figures. In Britain they were regarded as eccentrics who might happen to be geniuses.

In Italy, as in France, the term *ingenieri* is considered an honorific title, and many of the railways' best engineers were Italians. With the flair, the inventiveness, the love of improvization, the relish at coping with the unexpected typical of their countrymen, they grappled successfully with the appalling problems of providing a route, inevitably littered with long and tricky tunnels through very difficult terrain, down the mountainous Italian peninsula. Worst of all was the Cristina tunnel, one of the six needed to pass through the Apennines between Naples and Foggia. The soil was treacherous clay, which collapsed on the tunnellers frequently and unpredictably. In the end they had to excavate a deep trench filled with masonry before the timber supports for the tunnel itself could be installed.

But the greatest of all the Italian engineers was Germain Someiller, who was responsible for the tunnel under Mont Cenis, the first to carry a railway under the Alps. He devised the revolutionary pneumatic drill, which alone was capable of tunnelling through hard Alpine rocks, while also showing an unprecedented care for his workers, for whom he provided special villages – a marked contrast to the English contractors who had let

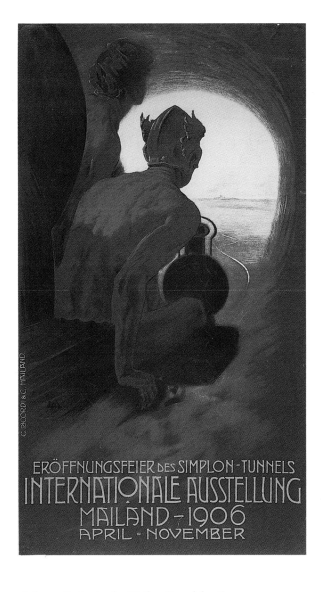

G. RICORDI & C. MAILAND

ERÖFFNUNGSFEIER DES SIMPLON-TUNNELS
INTERNATIONALE AUSSTELLUNG
MAILAND-1906
APRIL-NOVEMBER

A dramatic poster by Metlcovitx celebrating
the opening of the Simplon, one of the last
of the great railway tunnels under the Alps –
until the new ones are opened early next century.

their navvies freeze in the winter cold of the Pennines during the three years it took to dig the Woodhead tunnel between Sheffield and Manchester.

The Germans, too, had their unsung heroes, notably Wilhelm von Pressel, who was responsible for many of the lines in the Balkans and the Near East – and who died, impoverished and heart-broken, cursing the name of the financier, Baron Maurice von Hirsch, who had cheated him and made an enormous fortune out of his efforts. His lines were continued by Meissner Pasha, who built hundreds of miles of line from Damascus to Mecca through waterless deserts with a workforce of a dozen nationalities.

It was not only undeveloped countries which had to rely on foreign engineers. The first (but only the first) railways of virtually every country outside Britain were built by British contractors using British-built locomotives: when Thomas Brassey built the first major line outside Paris, to Rouen, his engineer, W. P. Buddicom, set up a locomotive factory in the town.

Labour-intensive: building the East Bengal Railway linking Calcutta with the outlying districts of Nadia and Far Idpur.

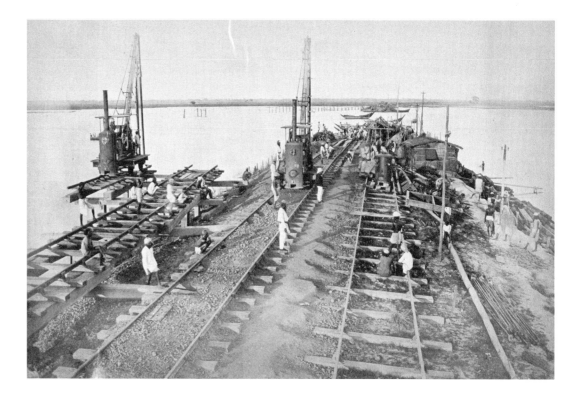

In Russia the first major line, between Moscow and St Petersburg, was built by George Washington Whistler, the father of the painter. But the Russians soon learnt to build as fast and, initially, as shoddily as the Americans. They, like everyone else, including even Brunel, was fully aware that a railway did not earn a penny until it was complete. And if this meant laying tracks on bare earth, so much the worse (one British contractor, George Pauling, used to forget about the bridges on his routes through Southern Africa: they could be built from the revenues from the original line, even if this meant ferrying passengers and freight across rivers in the wet seasons).

By the time they came to construct the Trans-Siberian railway, the Russians could rely on their own great engineers like Constantine Ya Mikhailovski, who built some of the line at the unbelievable rate of 3.2 km (2 miles) a day. But the greatest of all the Russian engineers was Alexander Yugovich, the 'deceptively dull-eyed' engineer who built the first Chinese Eastern Railway. According to Harmon Tupper (in *To The Great Ocean*) he and his colleagues had to cope simultaneously with 'deserts and mountain ranges, arctic cold, rampaging floods, pestilence, bandits, saboteurs, and obstructive officials', in a line over 900 miles (1450 km) long in which 'there were no utilizable labourers and fewer than six towns, each the periodic prey of Manchurian outlaws.' Unsurprisingly the roads between the few settlements were 'fantastically rough, and, during the rainy season, remained impassable until tediously filled in with brush and innumerable logs.'

There were other, equally remarkable, engineers whose names are now forgotten: George Totten, responsible for the railway across the Panama Peninsula, is commemorated only by a plaque at the end of the line. Perhaps the greatest achievement of all was the Central Trans-Andean, one of the wonders of the world, which rises to over 14,000 feet (4270 m), with a branch which climbs higher than Mont Blanc, a railway built through mountainous deserts where there was neither food, fodder nor water. Yet the name of the chief engineer, Ernesto Malinowski, is now forgotten, and his assistant, Martyn van Brocklin, is remembered, if at all, for a much lesser achievement as chief engineer of the El, New York's famous elevated railroad.

In the United States the long life of John B. Jervis, who died, aged ninety, in 1885 spanned and symbolized the development of the American railway network. Jervis started

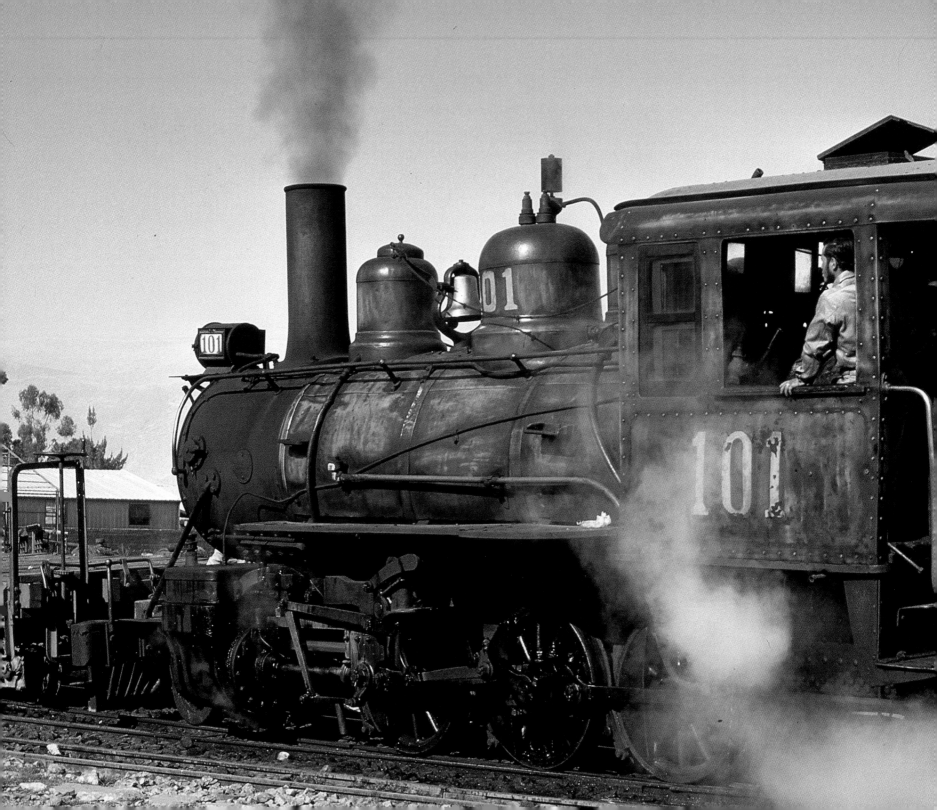

by learning his civil engineering working on the Delaware & Hudson Canal. After persuading the promoters of the first railways in New York State to use steam power rather than horse-drawn wagons he went on to develop what became known as the 'American-type' engine, the 4–4–0 design – with four small wheels on a swivel (a 'bogie') guiding the four driving wheels behind and making the whole flexible enough for the sharp curves normal on most American railroads. He then went west, helping the New York Central to complete its route to Chicago, then spent seven years extending the Rock Island Line west across the Mississippi – and helping a little-known railroad lawyer, Abraham Lincoln, to defend the company's right to bridge the river against the onslaughts (physical as well as legal) mounted by the well-entrenched maritime interests.

*B*ehind the first generation of engineers, particularly the British ones, were the contractors. For thirty years these were not merely the builders they are today, but the prototype of great industrial entrepreneurs – except that the businesses created by men like Thomas Brassey and Sir Samuel Morton Peto were strictly personal, they had no successors. They, like the great engineers, were stars, men who had risen far, often from humble roots, for railways were enormously important democratizing influences in the important sense that anyone could climb to fame and fortune by demonstrating outstanding skill or cunning, however lowly their origins, which is one of the reasons why they attracted such a disproportionate number of able people.

The most typical example was Sir Samuel Morton Peto. He had risen to fame as a builder (of the Houses of Parliament and the Reform Club, amongst other major achievements) before he became one of the country's leading contractors, and one of the few with the reputation of caring for his employees. His reputation was enhanced during the Crimean War when a gang of navvies under his instructions built a crucial railway from Sebastopol to Balaklava in record time after the Army's own engineers had made a hash of the project. He was promptly awarded a baronetcy and soon became a leading nonconformist member of the House of Commons.

Even a shunting engine – like this one in the little town of Huancayo in the Peruvian Andes – can embody the magic of steam travel.

But despite his genuine public service he, like his fellows, was treated with the normal English attitude towards *nouveaux riches*. They suffered a steady stream of vituperation, of contempt for their sometimes rough manners and their insufficiently respectful attitude towards the established political system and the honours it bestowed: when Thomas Brassey, the greatest of them all, was awarded a decoration by the Emperor of Austria, he simply said 'Thank you, Mrs Brassey will enjoy it.'

Not surprisingly they were thought particularly disrespectful in their attitude to the House of Commons, in which many of them bought seats – though few used them to as much purpose as Peto. Despite Peto's reputation, Anthony Trollope painted a highly libellous portrait of him in *Dr Thorne*. He was only lightly disguised as Sir Roger Scatcherd, whom Trollope described as a 'whilom drunken stone-mason in Barchester' who was 'elevated for the moment to the dizzy pinnacle of a newspaper hero' because of 'some highly necessary bit of railway to be made in half the time that such work would properly demand' – a sneering reference to Peto's achievement in the Crimea. But in Trollope's eyes the mere fact that such work would demand 'great means and courage as well' did not offset Scatcherd's other failings, including, one suspects, his failure to be well-born.

But the contractors' very success limited their future. By 1852 Britain already had the railway system which still serves it well today. For another decade they promoted what were called 'contractors' lines', railways whose ostensible purpose was to fill in the gaps of the earlier network or to provide competition for existing lines, but which, too often, were simple 'make work' for the promoter. But their fall came through the attempts made by companies like the London, Chatham and South Coast to extend existing railway lines into the City. The enormous sums required led directly to the worst financial 'smash' (the contemporary term) seen in the whole crash-ridden century, the Overend Gurney scandal of 1866. This wiped out a whole generation of entrepreneurs and contractors. The most distinguished victim was Peto, who managed to pay his debts, but was forced to flee abroad after a vicious campaign of press harassment led by the *Daily Telegraph*.

As a result they had to look outside Britain for work. Abroad they had a mixed reputation. Thomas Brassey spread the reputation of the Briton as a truly honest man wherever he went. But, in general, the breed acquired the reputation accorded a century

later to British football hooligans by the activities of the less scrupulous of his fellows –
notably John Sadleir, the model for Charles Dickens' character Merdle. The original
cheated the Swedes so thoroughly that the country promptly and permanently abandoned the whole idea of privately-developed railways.

So the breed died out, to be replaced by men who were more purely contractors in
the modern sense. The only other countries where they flourished were Canada,
and, more surprisingly, Russia. In Canada, indeed, it was two outstanding showmen-
entrepreneurs, William Mackenzie and Donald Mann, who induced the government to
build the ill-fated rival to the Canadian Pacific, the lines which were later merged and
nationalized as the Canadian National Railway.

In Russia the entrepreneurs were opportunists, less involved in the fabric of national
life than in Anglo-Saxon countries. As J. A. Westwood described them in his *History of
Russian Railways* they included men:

> . . . who had entered the railway field after making their fortunes in other business, men like
> Bernardaki who became a promoter after making his fortune in the Siberian liquor trade;
> professional bankers who simply became chairmen of the railways they were financing, and
> then a new generation which made its fortune solely from railway promotion.

They were a mixed bunch. There was Von Derviz, whose opportunity was given him by
an old school chum who became Minister of Finance – and who eventually retired to
Italy and built an opera house where performances were staged solely for his own personal
delectation. The most improbable Russian success story in what was a profoundly anti-
Semitic society was that of Polyakov, a Jewish former plasterer who was responsible for
many of the country's major lines.

In the United States by the end of the century the most typical figure in the business
was the builder-contractor. Employed by the financiers who dominated the railway
world, they lacked the entrepreneurial independence of the Petos and Brasseys, but were
none the less remarkable for all that.

The archetype was George Pauling, who, like all his kind, was a roving entrepreneur,
ready for any business, from selling a ready-made mixture of whisky and water in Jordan
to mining for gold and diamonds in South Africa, where he found that building railways

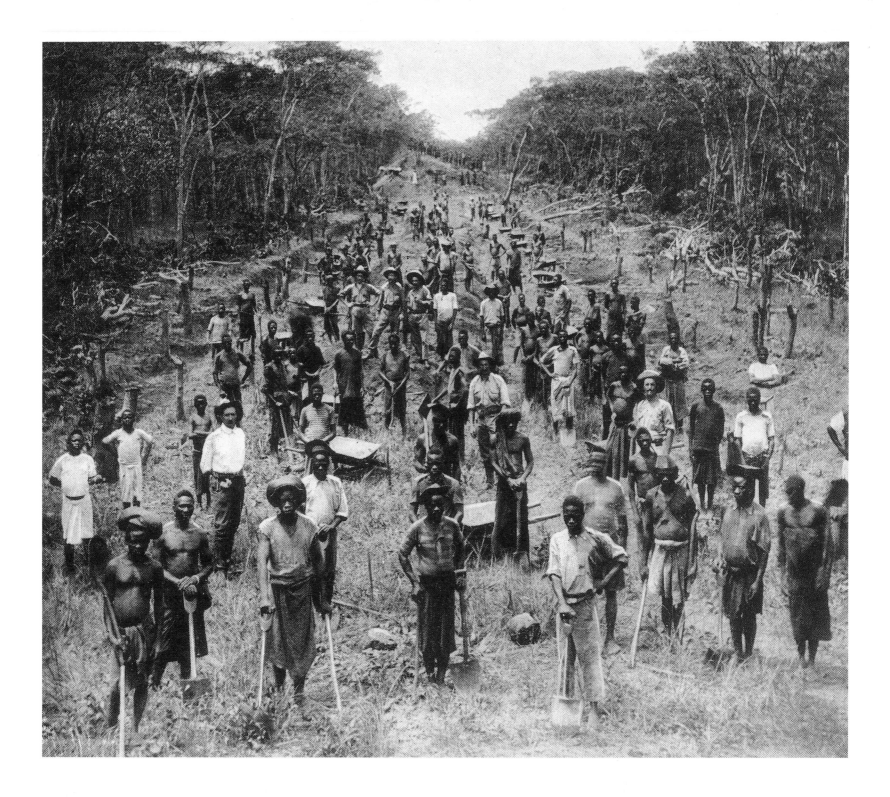

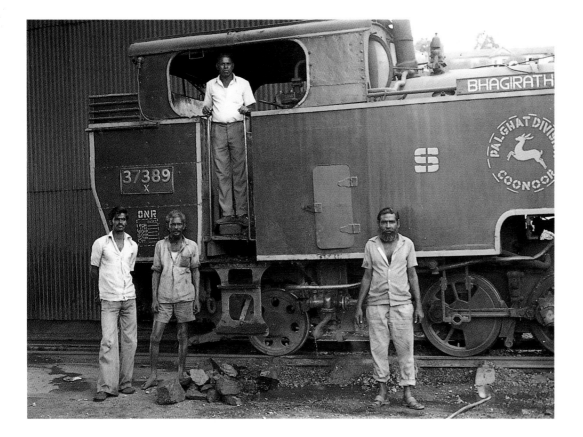

These Indian railwaymen at Ootacamund, in Tamil Nadhu province, have the same dignity as their counterparts the world over.

provided the best outlet for his talents. These included an infallible eye for the lie of the land and the most economic route for a railway, a quality common to all such engineers and contractors, and one which Pauling exploited by negotiating contracts on the basis of the promoters' original plans, for he was, usually rightly, confident of additional profits by finding a better and shorter route. Like his fellows Pauling had incredible stamina, and an even more unbelievable capacity for food and drink – he and two friends once downed a thousand oysters at a sitting, and drank three hundred bottles of 'excellent and refreshing' German beer while stuck for a couple of days on the Beira railway in south-west Africa.

Opposite A horde of locals, a few white supervisors, a typical scene anywhere outside Europe – in fact they were preparing the way for the proposed line from the Cape to Cairo.

3 Capitalists and Workers

I n his essay on railway emigrants Robert Louis Stevenson reflected that 'all this epochal turmoil [the first American transcontinental railroad] was conducted by gentlemen in frockcoats and with a view to nothing more extraordinary than a fortune and a subsequent visit to Paris.' RLS's 'men in frockcoats' were financiers who flourished as never before thanks to the railways' insatiable appetite for capital – which obviously offered equally unprecedented opportunities for capital gain.

Naturally American railroads, the largest system, owned since the beginning by private companies, formed (and still form) the best example of the interreaction of railways and capitalism, and a fascinating clash it has proved over the past hundred and fifty years.

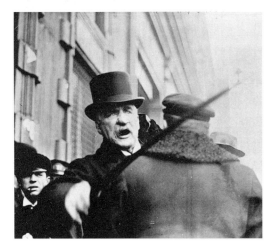

Capitalism in action. J. P. Morgan didn't like press photographers – would you if you had a nose as obtrusive as his?

In their early days the American railroads attracted more than their fair share of chancers, since for half a century or more they were 'the biggest game in town'. As a result the railway tycoons became synonymous with capitalist greed. But their opponents never tried to reconcile the villains' supposedly evil nature with the legacy they left: the world's finest railway system. For few if any of the early railroad magnates were as purely destructive as their modern equivalents, the band of financiers who in the 1960s despoiled Penn Central, the result of the merger of two systems, the Pennsylvania and the New York Central, which had once been the pride of the American railroad system, as fine as any tracks in the world.

Of course the first generation did include shady financiers, like Dr Durant, the evil genius of the Union Pacific, but more typical were the Big Four – Leland Stanford, Mark Hopkins, Henry Huntingdon and Charles Crocker – who financed and built the Central Pacific, the western third of the first transcontinental railroad system. Having pledged

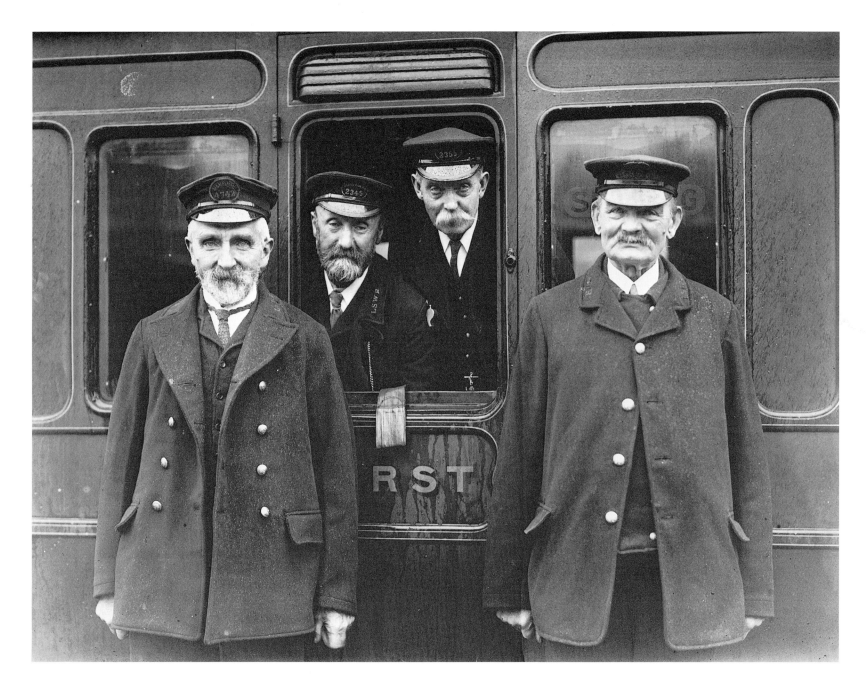

The railway tradition. On Christmas Eve 1920 these four veterans retired from the London & South Western (the line from London to Southampton) with 207 years service between them.

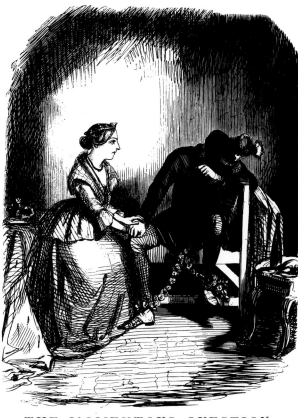

Punch – then a decidedly radical weekly – assumed, rightly, that even the mightiest in the land were caught up in the railway mania of 1845–46.

THE MOMENTOUS QUESTION.

"Tell me, oh tell me, dearest Albert, have *you* any Railway Shares?"

their all, and risked bankruptcy over a period of years in the face of the systematic indifference, indeed the total hostility, of their fellow capitalists, they naturally felt entitled to the spoils once the railroad was built. Equally naturally, their assumption that their daring had earned them the right to govern California, the state they had linked to the rest of the country, as they thought fit bred a deep-rooted resentment among its inhabitants. Yet today their names are associated less with their former despotism than with memorials to their generosity, from Stanford University to the Huntingdon Memorial Library.

The most typical railway tycoon was Jay Gould. For a generation he cast an atmosphere of terror around him. 'When Jay Gould was in his prime,' ran the doggerel, 'all the other railroad magnates were wondering which tree to climb.' But, unlike other tycoons, notably John D. Rockefeller, he never went in for elaborate and expensive public relations gestures, and unlike one of his rivals, Jim Fisk, he had no exotic mistress to captivate the New Yorkers. Gould's neglect of public opinion meant that newspapers concentrated their hostility on to him – a bias which misled later researchers who relied too heavily on such sources. At the time, explains his great-grandson Kingdon Gould Jr, he capitalized on newspaper rumours: 'if it were reported that he were buying shares, instead he'd be selling shares.' Kingdon Gould excused his ancestor as being 'the last boy on the block, who came from a very poor rural family in upstate New York. By the time he arrived on the business scene, the Astors; the Vanderbilts, Rockefellers, the Harrimans were well-established families of great power.'

Indeed his financial habits were no better and no worse than his contemporaries'. Moreover he genuinely cared for the systems he plotted so deviously to control. As Kingdon Gould says: 'He was very much into the details of how a line was being operated … he endeavoured to obtain cargo for the railroad.' His enemies said that this was merely to boost the line's profits for long enough to enable him to sell his stock. But behind his manoeuvrings was a dream, one he shared with that other railroad genius E. H. Harriman, of creating the first transcontinental network, a never-realized dream which could have been of enormous benefit to the whole United States.

Not that Gould was averse to some splendidly devious financial manoeuvres. In the course of one battle between his Erie Railroad and Commodore Vanderbilt's New York Central both sides kept lowering the rates for carrying boxcars full of cattle. In the end Gould threw in the towel and allowed his rival to keep all the traffic at a mere $1 a boxcar. According to Kingdon Gould: 'It was only later that it was discovered that Gould had bought as many cattle as he possibly could and was shipping them on Vanderbilt's railroad to the eastern markets at the ludicrously low fare he had forced his rival to charge.'

The tycoons' battles naturally spread to the judicial system. The business historian John Steele Gordon relates how everyone in New York had to have their own judge, in case of emergency. Politicians were also part of the system. When both Gould and Commodore Vanderbilt were bribing the New York State legislature in the Erie Railroad affair, Gould arrived in Albany (the state capital) with a suitcase full of thousand dollar bills and was handing them out very liberally. But, alas for the legislators, once Commodore Vanderbilt decided to withdraw, 'the legislature was furious because suddenly their votes weren't worth any money anymore.'

The Goulds, the Vanderbilts and their like were operating in markets which they themselves had done much to create, and not only in New York. Within fifteen years of the opening of the Liverpool & Manchester Railway, England was in the throes of an unprecedented mania for railway investment. Everyone with any money became involved, from the Brontë sisters who invested their meagre savings in the Yorkshire & Midland Railway, to the worldly Charles Greville, the Clerk to the Privy Council, even though he had been warned off by no less a personage than the Governor of the Bank of England.

The demand for capital from countries the world over solidified the City of London's central position in the world's financial scene from that day on, providing a market big enough for all comers to be accommodated – at a price. The stocks and bonds issued by railway companies dominated the City from the 1840s to the 1890s. But the London market was already well established before the railways arrived. In New York the Wall Street market was largely the creation of the railways and their insatiable demand for finance, although they were not the first large-scale borrowers. In the words of John Steele Gordon:

In 1861 the United States government owed around $63 million, by the end of the Civil War they owed 2\frac{1}{2}$ billion. And virtually all of that money was raised on Wall Street ... in 1860 Wall Street was a small market, by 1865 it was second only to London ... railroads were more important than the Federal government because they continued, whereas the government immediately began reducing its debt after the Civil War and by the end of the century had almost eliminated it.

By the late 1860s New Yorkers were involved in their own equivalent of the railway mania which had seized the English twenty years earlier. John Steele Gordon explains how

> ... for the first time people who had nothing to do with finance became involved in speculation. Women were coming down from uptown and standing in line in brokerage houses in order to take a gamble on railroad stocks. Clergymen were gambling on railroad stocks. The lunch counter, the first fast food restaurant in the world, was invented in New York in the early 1860s because people didn't have time to go back home for lunch.

Gene Proudfit, a retired railroad executive with a long memory, explains: 'Many of the investors were from the United Kingdom, from the Netherlands, from Germany. And these resources always centred on New York. And to a certain extent the banks or the financial institutions controlled what the railroads did.'

But in the 1890s at least one tycoon escaped their clutches:

> In the case of the Union Pacific, Mr Harriman developed resources on his own initiative, bypassing the banks, because he didn't want to be controlled by the New York bankers. And for many, many years a large block of Union Pacific stock was held by the Netherlands.

*F*or all their financially dubious habits the early tycoons left another legacy. The great railway systems, especially in Britain and the United States, were the first modern businesses, relying on increasingly elaborate and pioneering management techniques. Originally they had been run like armies, which were the only other organizations of such size spread over so broad a canvas. For the same good reasons, many railway systems throughout the world were dominated by former military men, and remained subject to a military-type hierarchy, if only because their successful operation depended on imposing discipline on a workforce which was strung out over hundreds, sometimes thousands, of miles of track.

The military atmosphere was noted early on. For the opening of the Liverpool & Manchester 'orders of the day' were issued to participants. Subsequent railway workers were 'in the service': they reported for duty and had to stay by their posts until relieved. Leave – even today railwaymen do not have holidays – required written permission. But the railways went further than the armies, since their role was permanent – unlike soldiers railwaymen were fighting all day and every day, 365 days a year.

The same factors applied while the railways were under construction, as Jim Ehrenberger, a retired railroad worker, points out, when the first transcontinental railroad was being built in the years immediately after the Civil War.

> The generals they had in the Civil War also came and operated the construction camps. They had people who knew how to organize the supplies . . . and I think it was the military that ensured that the first transcontinental railroad was built as quickly as it was!

(It was opened just four years after the end of the war.) The same talents were required once the railways were in operation, says Ehrenberger.

> It's almost impossible to operate the railroad like you would a factory where there could be a supervisor overseeing one operation. A railroad is not like a factory where everything is under one roof. The railroad is actually a factory without walls. [So you needed a military-type management system] . . . in order to have everyone understand what they were supposed to do, when they were supposed to do it, and how they were supposed to do it. As a result railway management procedures the world over were codified in immense volumes, which were treated as holy writ.

Indeed they were far more militaristic in organization than even the most disciplined army, which inevitably allows (and often has to rely on) a certain degree of initiative from even the smallest unit. By contrast the railways depended from their inception on a tradition of total adherence to orders, which was most crucial at the lowest operating level.

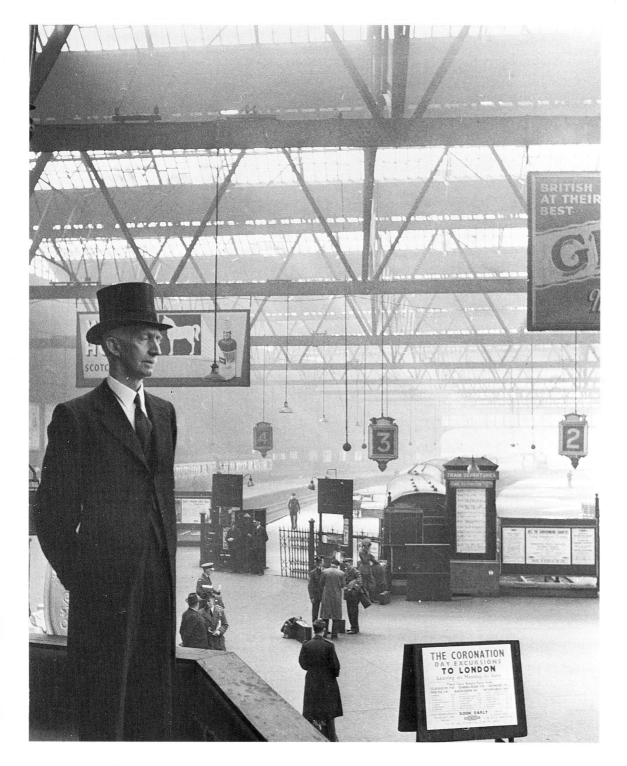

Not so long ago: Robert J. Buchanan, Station Master at Princes Street Station in Edinburgh waiting to receive The Queen and the Duke of Edinburgh on their way to the Coronation.

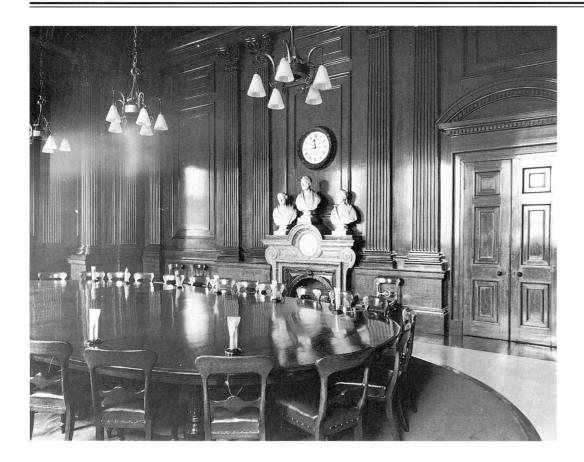

The boardroom of the London & North Western Railway Company at Euston. The company, and the room, set a style which lasted for a century or more.

The militaristic tradition was stronger outside the United States. In Prussia the railwaymen's uniforms were almost indistinguishable from those worn by soldiers, and for a long time station staff had to stand to attention when trains passed through. In Britain, before the railways bred their own, the army had naturally furnished the early managers – most famously Captain Mark Huish, the autocratic general manager of the London & North Western, the world's first major railway network. In France, by contrast, the Polytechnique and other Grandes Ecoles produced an abundance of officers trained and ready to command any major enterprise. They naturally took the management of the country's railways in their stride. The United States had no reserve of officers or industrial

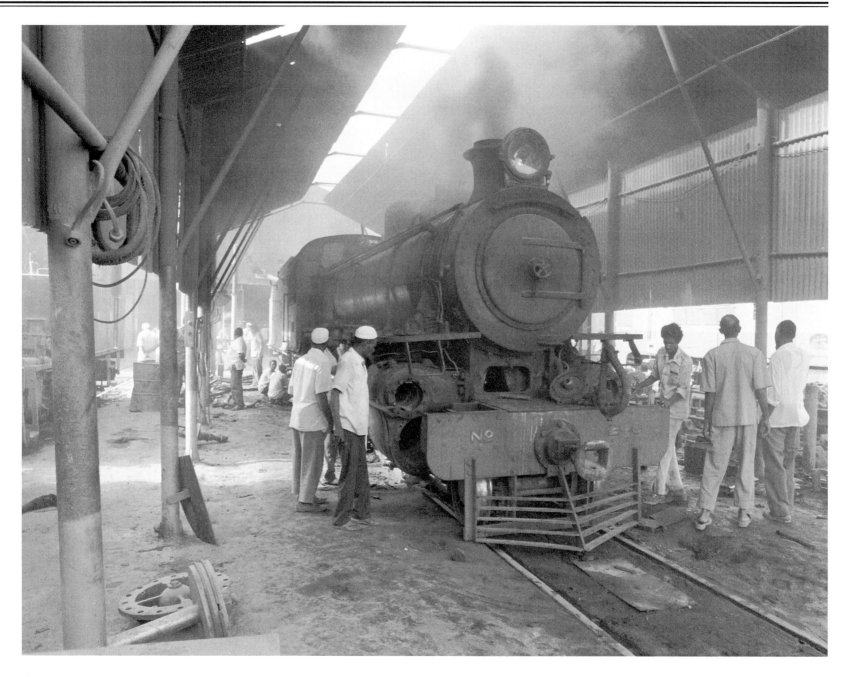

technocrats so had to breed its own, men who soon emerged as the pioneers of modern industrial management. Alfred Chandler was perfectly justified in entitling his book on the subject *Railroads, the Nation's First Big Business*. For the railways' bosses were not only the most important managers of their age, they were the models for tycoons in other industries. Andrew Carnegie, creator of the modern American steel industry, openly admitted that his hero was Tom Scott of the Pennsylvania Railroad, where Carnegie himself made his name as a telegraph operator early in his career.

The admiration was not surprising, for the mighty 'Pennsy' had gone the furthest in developing modern-style management systems. The Baltimore and Ohio had been the first company to separate the financial from operating functions, and this improvement was followed by Daniel C. McCallum of the New York Central (later, as we will see in Chapter 4, the man who did most to exploit the advantages possessed by the Union's railroad system during the Civil War) who laid out a modern-style organizational pattern, including an unprecedented clarity in defining the roles of different departments. But it was the Pennsy, first under J. Edgar Thomson and then under Tom Scott, which brought together all these experiences into a coherent whole.

Railways were totally different from any of their contemporary business organizations. First, and crucially, they were the prototype of the modern corporation, run by professional managers, who did not necessarily control the company's shares. As John Steele Gordon puts it:

> There had never been a case before where the people who ran the company day to day were not the owners ... Moreover, with a factory you can shut it down until demand picks up ... but with a railroad, which is anyway highly capital-intensive ... you have to keep to a regular schedule, which means that the train runs whether it's empty or full. And for this reason railroads often operate below cost, because they have to.

As he points out they were also

> ... the only big business the average person encountered on a daily basis ... the great big manufacturing corporations were in many respects an abstraction ... but they took the train every morning to get to work and when the train didn't come, they were annoyed at the railroads ... they were day-to-day life.

Opposite *A Pacific steam locomotive of Sudan Railways in the workshops at Atbara – more like this would have prevented the starvation in the south of the country.*

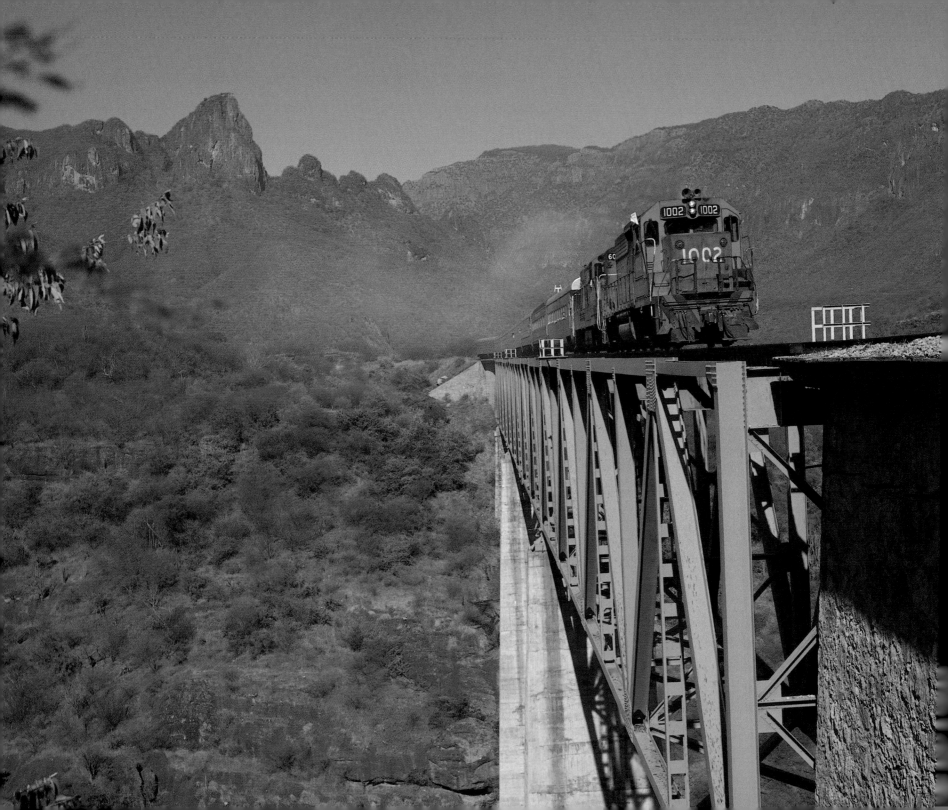

As a result they naturally attracted more than their fair share of unfavourable attention. As early as 1846 the philosopher Herbert Spencer prefigured a seemingly modern complaint, the dominance of corporations, especially the bigger ones, by managers and major shareholders at the expense of smaller shareholders. He was also referring to railway companies when he observed that 'corporate conscience is ever inferior to the individual conscience – that a body of men will commit as a joint act, that which every individual of them would shrink from did he feel individually responsible.'

For even the managers of the great railroad systems wielded enormous power. In the words of the historian Lord Bryce:

> Railroad kings are amongst the greatest men, perhaps I may say the greatest men in America. They have power, more power – that is more opportunity in making their will prevail – than perhaps anyone in political life, except the president and the speaker who after all hold theirs only for four years and two years while the railroad monarch may keep his for life.

But it was also a business within which the humblest employee could, and often did, rise to the top. Although the directors of railway companies were usually grandees nominated by the City, or Wall Street (or, in continental Europe, by the government) there was plenty of room for promotion through the ranks to become the general managers or superintendents who wielded the actual day-to-day power. This applied even to former radicals like the executive who wrote his memoirs, *A General Manager's Story*, under the name of Herbert Hamblen. After many adventures, and many tales of the appalling way railroad companies treated their employees, he ended his working life as a general manager calling in strike-breakers when the railwaymen demanded increased wages. The strike broken, he could note smugly, 'I flatter myself that today our stock compares favourably with the best in the market.'

*T*he power of the railroads, and their bosses, was bound to breed a reaction. The first was the so-called Granger movement in the American mid-west, a populist revolt by the farmers against the railroads' abuse of their monopoly power to transport grain to market. By that time the only organized industrial force powerful enough to confront the railroads was Standard Oil, an even more unified and formidable monopoly. Moreover

Opposite Even diesel engines can be romantic beasts in the right setting – as here on the Chinipas Bridge, the highest on the Chihuahua Pacific Railway in Mexico.

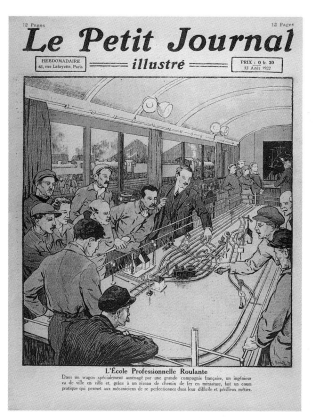

L'École Professionnelle Roulante
Dans un wagon spécialement aménagé par une grande compagnie française, un ingénieur va de ville en ville et, grâce à un réseau de chemin de fer en miniature, fait un cours pratique qui permet aux mécaniciens de se perfectionner dans leur difficile et périlleux métier.

French railwaymen, amongst the most professional in the world, learning their trade on a model track.

'The Standard' had a weapon denied to the railroads' other customers: it could move its oil through pipelines. Other companies which were at the mercy of the railroad sympathized with the Grangers and the railroads' other opponents, for they felt equally powerless.

By the late 1880s the country's first regulatory body, the Interstate Commerce Commission (ICC) was set up. Yet, as Frank Wilner, a railroad lobbyist, points out:

> It was the railroads that wanted the legislation. They were concerned that there would be cutthroat competition and that rates would fall and profits would fall. So they took their power to Washington and demanded regulation in the hope that it would create a floor beneath which rates wouldn't fall ... rather than what the Populists expected, a ceiling above which rates wouldn't rise.

But, within a generation, the system had hardened, had ensured a mediocre uniformity.

> Railroads were no longer in charge of their own destiny. They were unable to go to a customer and design a package exclusively for him. And as regulation evolved over the years, the regulators insisted on an average rate for an average customer. But in fact there were no such things as average customers.

Moreover, Wilner continues, 'If there were two railroads competing from here to there, both of these had to have the same rate. As a result price was no longer a means of competition. And it took entrepreneurship out of the railroads.' As he says, top railway managers tended to be either engineers, interested only in operating the railroads, or lawyers, familiar with the regulatory jungle in Washington.

> They knew nothing about customers or designing a package. The result was that railroads were run for the convenience of the railroad operating department and the customer was never considered. Well all it took was a competing mode and it was the trucks ... Truckers were run by small businessmen. They perhaps ran one or two trucks. They understood that quality is whatever the customer says it is ... So those who wanted a faster delivery rate, or those who wanted a lower rate, or some other very specific service, found themselves going to trucks.

Moreover, as the veteran railroad analyst Isabel Benham points out, the regulatory mechanism became a marvellous excuse for the railroads. When she first worked on Wall Street in the early 1930s: 'about one-third of the railroad mileage was in bankruptcy ... they blamed their situation on the government because the government was helping with highways' – although the Depression was more to blame than the government.

For all their steadily diminishing power, the railroads remained the symbol of ruthless, exploitative monopoly capitalism. A whole generation of 'muckrakers', culminating in Matthew Josephson, whose influential book *The Robber Barons* was published as late as 1932, painted the railroad tycoons as purely evil figures. Yet it is not the tycoons who were the real villains of the piece but the politicians who demanded the money at times when the promoters were either financially hard-pressed, or saw no reason to shell out, or both. The greed was not confined to the United States, politicians were just as bad in Canada. In his autobiography Sir Edmund Hornby, a British businessman disgusted by the Canadian way of doing business, wrote how 'as usual it was a Psalm-singing Protestant Dissenter who, holding seven or eight votes in the palm of his hand, volunteered to do the greasing job for a consideration'; yet the country's pioneering transcontinental railway, the Canadian Pacific, was built and operated with exemplary honesty.

The unpopularity of the railway kings in the United States resulted in the glamorization of common criminals who were treated as popular heroes. Frank and Jesse James were sheltered from their pursuers for several years because their opponents were railway companies. In *The Story of American Railroads* Stewart Holbrook explains how 'farmers who felt they had been cheated ... other men who had lost their savings in wild-cat railroad stocks and bonds ... laboring men who felt the railroads were grinding them down were not going to help the strike-breaking "Pinkertons" to hunt them down.' This feeling foreshadowed attitudes towards another unpopular group, the agents who later tried to enforce Prohibition.

*I*n the United States the railroads' operations came to be rigidly controlled, not only by the federal government, but also by the unions. This, again, was a legacy of the early days when the tycoons treated their employees as mere fodder – although we

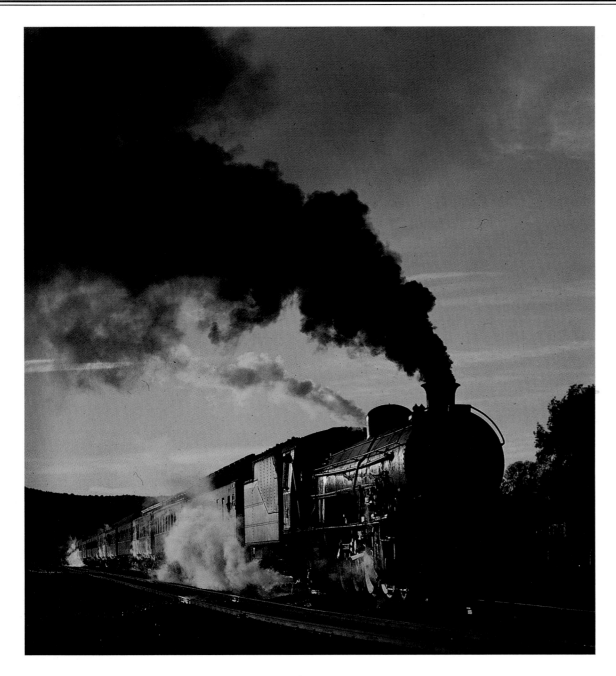

A scarcity of oil, cheap coal and long distance hauls made steam haulage economically viable in South Africa long after it had been abandoned elsewhere.

should not be misled into thinking that railwaymen were different from other workers: it is merely that we know more about them. Railways, like airlines today, had such an aura of glamour that their every activity was far more open to the glare of publicity than smaller, more humdrum industries.

But the railwaymen did indeed have a case. In the United States, as elsewhere in the world, their hours were long – working literally days at a stretch and twelve hours without food were normal. Many of the jobs were appallingly dangerous, and in the absence of any industrial legislation the companies were mostly indifferent to the fates of their 'servants'. Herbert Hamblen tells how one innocent railwayman: 'believed that "accidents were largely due to the recklessness of the men themselves . . ." Poor fellow! He was blown from the top of his train a few months afterwards, and found by the section gang, frozen stiff.'

Worst off were the brakemen who had to couple the cars together – the American railroads opposed automatic links until well into the present century. Hence the accuracy of the bitter ballad:

> *'Twas only a poor dying brakeman,*
> *Simply a hard lab'ring man . . .*
> *'Twas only a poor mangled being,*
> *Nobody knew "What's his name".*

This was only a slight exaggeration. As Horace Herr wrote in *The Railroad Man's Magazine* in 1910:

Dan watched a gang of boomer [itinerant] brakemen and switchmen come in the yards and ask for work. The yardmaster asked them to hold up their hands in lieu of references. If the applicants had several fingers missing, the yardmaster knew they were 'old timers' and would be able to go on the job as experienced workers and not as students.

The dangers were increased by cost-cutting managements, and reductions in wages were met by the response, reported by Hamblen, that because of 'the exorbitant wages you men are receiving the railroad would be placed in the hands of a receiver.' A guard is quoted by Cyril B. Andrews in *The Railway Age* as saying

In my early days we were called brakesmen; we had no brake vans; we had to ride on the top of the carriages or on the loaded vans, anywhere we could, and to get on and off anyhow we could. And on a frosty night it was getting off. Our limbs were often benumbed with cold; we were sometimes so stiff with cold that we had to be lifted off, and some, when they were lifted off, were found to be frozen to death.

As a result of their experiences the railwaymen were linked (and separated from the community as a whole) by bonds which have lasted until today, making them a proud, hierarchical, introverted, skilled, conservative group. Like the navvies they produced their own language, their own folklore, their own language, their own songs. As Frank McKenna put it in *The Railway Workers, 1840–1970* they were 'a new form of industrial anthropology, a tribalistic grouping of men based on an elaborate division of labour, a hierarchy of groups and a ritualistic adherence to territory, myth symbolism and insignia unknown outside the specified boundaries.'

In the United States the railwaymen organized themselves, not into unions, but into 'Brotherhoods'. The name may seem quaint today, but in the nineteenth century it meant precisely what it said. The 'boomers' in particular often relied on their paid-up membership card in a railway brotherhood. In the words of Freeman Hubbard in *Pennsylvania Songs and Legends*: 'During his frequent lean periods he would shove this under the nose of a worthy brother when he wanted to eat, sleep, ride or all three, and it usually achieved the desired result.'

Because railways were the biggest, most ruthless and best organized of industries, and because of the solidarity of their employees, they inevitably featured in some of the most famous early strikes, especially in the United States. The first major struggle came in the bad years of the 1870s when wages were constantly being reduced. The employers were alert to the slightest sign of disturbance, for they had been scared stiff by the horrors they associated with the Paris Commune of 1870–71, and were obsessed with the effects of 'foreign agitators' on their workforce. By no coincidence Eugene Debs, the symbol of American radical unionism, first rose to fame as the head of the American Railway Union. This obsession with an 'alien' or, later, 'Communist' infection was to remain a recurring theme in American history until the collapse of the Soviet Union at the end of the 1980s.

A great wave of strikes in 1877 shocked the bosses but provided a precedent for a future theme: the federal government, while by no means 'progressive,' was more inclined to act as mediator, less hostile to the strikers than the railroad magnates. Even President Hayes, supposedly a creature of the railroads, wrote in his diary that: 'The railroad strikers, as a rule, are good men, sober, intelligent and industrious.'

The combination of militancy, itself a product of bitter early experiences, and the strict hierarchy of railroad unions, an inheritance of the militaristic railway tradition, had a fatal effect on American railroads. Les Orear, a retired trade-unionist and railway historian, emphasizes how

> . . . the railroad labour scene was very fragmented . . . broken into many different unions, each
> with its own function . . . the engineers would be in one union, and the conductors would
> be in another, and the flagmen, the switchmen would be in another one and the telegraphers
> in another one . . . on and on it went . . . and they would hardly speak to each other.

This fragmentation gave the unions a considerable motive to resist change since the abolition of a given function would mean the end of a whole union. In the words of Isabel Benham, once diesel traction was introduced:

> . . . there was no need for a fireman in the cab of a locomotive. But it was twenty years or
> more before all the firemen were gotten off the railroad locomotives because the firemen had
> tenure on that particular job and legislation couldn't change that tenure . . . The railroad train
> had to have a caboose on the end and there was a conductor back there. And when they got
> the caboose off the railroad . . . yet the conductor stayed, because he had tenure.

The union's power was solidified in the First World War when the railroads were, effectively, operated by the government. As Gene Proudfit explains,

> They abolished the piece-work method of paying for services rendered and adopted an eight-
> hour day for employees in general. The exception was the operating brotherhoods where a
> hundred miles or eight hours was an eight-hour day. The hundred miles represented an
> eight-hour day at the time that they burned wood and the fireman fired by hand. Today
> in a diesel locomotive on the same premise a crew could make three days' pay in three and
> a half hours.

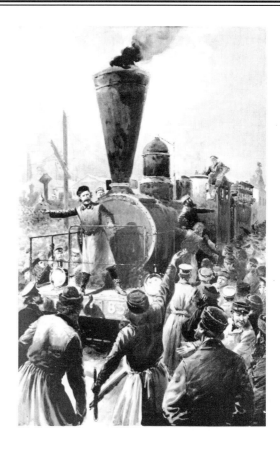

Revolution on the tracks: but these strikers holding up a train near Moscow in November 1905 were not to know that their efforts would be in vain – for the time being.

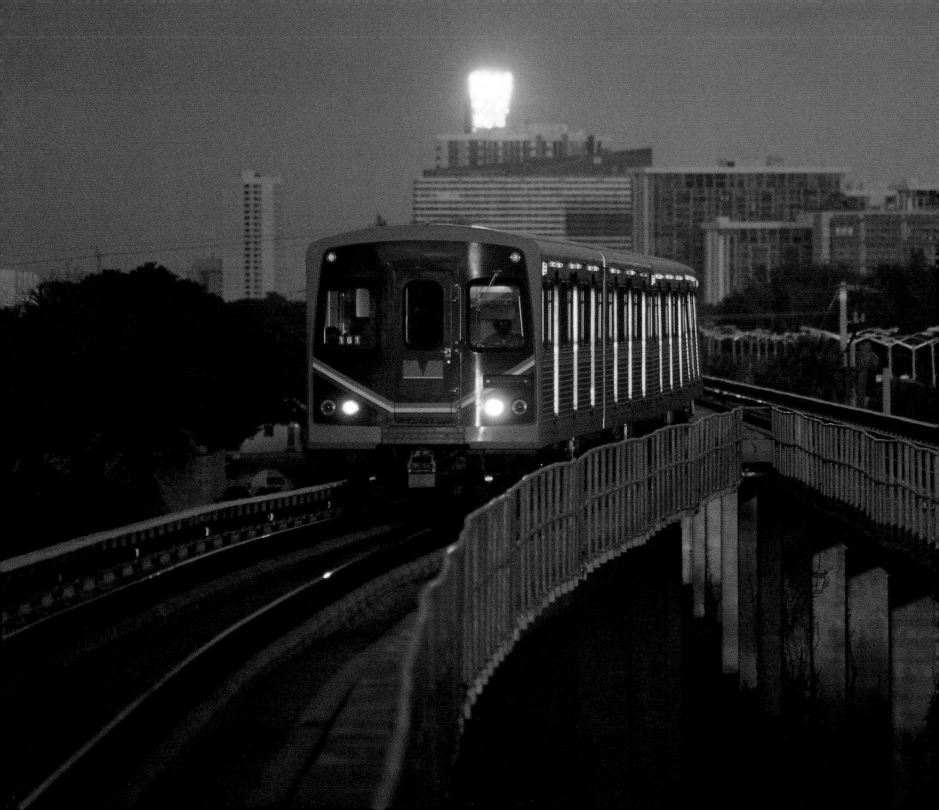

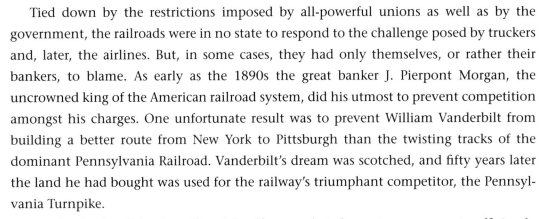

Tied down by the restrictions imposed by all-powerful unions as well as by the government, the railroads were in no state to respond to the challenge posed by truckers and, later, the airlines. But, in some cases, they had only themselves, or rather their bankers, to blame. As early as the 1890s the great banker J. Pierpont Morgan, the uncrowned king of the American railroad system, did his utmost to prevent competition amongst his charges. One unfortunate result was to prevent William Vanderbilt from building a better route from New York to Pittsburgh than the twisting tracks of the dominant Pennsylvania Railroad. Vanderbilt's dream was scotched, and fifty years later the land he had bought was used for the railway's triumphant competitor, the Pennsylvania Turnpike.

But the final nail in the railroads' coffin was that the systems were not sufficiently integrated. For all their size they were simply not big enough to provide the sort of nationwide service demanded by their customers. Although the major railroad systems, and above all the tycoons who controlled them, were attacked for their megalomania, there is a strong case to be made that their systems weren't big enough, that not even Jay Gould or Edward Harriman ever realized their dream of controlling a single system across the entire United States, with all the economic benefits this implied. As it was, the old saying that 'a hog can travel through Chicago without changing trains, but a passenger can't' remained true for a century until the effective demise of long-distance railroad travel in the 1960s and 1970s.

By 1981, when the Staggers Act finally freed the railroads from nearly a hundred years of restrictions, and they were again allowed to emerge, to charge what they wanted and to tighten up their operations, they had been reduced to a sad state, averaging under 20 mph (30 kph), less than a hundred years earlier. But, as we shall see in Chapter 10, the 1980s were the start of a new era for American railroads, as they were for most of the world's other rail systems.

The stuff of contemporary urban railway mythology:
an elevated railway in Miami.

4   *The War Machines*

The idea that railways were inevitably progressive, democratic, was given a rude response when they proved a godsend to governments, democratic or authoritarian, trying to tighten their grip. The authorities, even in democratic Britain, soon found them exceedingly useful in suppressing domestic discontent by rushing troops to the scene of any troublesome uprisings, In the 1830s and early 1840s the British government used them to carry troops to disturbances threatened by the Irish and by the revolutionary Chartists (who demanded such absurdities as universal adult suffrage).

The British experience was used by the Austrian promoter, Albrecht Gerstner, in his attempt to promote a network of lines throughout European Russia. The Tsar sat up and started to take an interest in the subject for the first time during the presentation when Gerstner told him:

> Your Majesty, at a notice of but twenty-four hours the railway will be able to transport five thousand infantry and five thousand cavalry with all their horses, cannons and wagons. Permit me to recall England's experience. There, during the recent Irish troubles, the government within two hours brought troops over the rail from Manchester to Liverpool, thence to be embarked for Dublin.

By 1848 his brother monarchs had used railways to move troops to put down the uprisings which shook Europe that year. By the early 1860s the Tsar had discovered that a mobile reserve of troops could save manpower previously tied up in border garrisons.

But it was the Indian Mutiny in 1857 which provided the most conclusive proof of the railways' usefulness in times of civil disorder. Such few lines as there were proved

Opposite Cattle trucks were good enough for this group of Royal Engineers on a narrow-gauge railway at Arras in France on the Western Front in World War I.

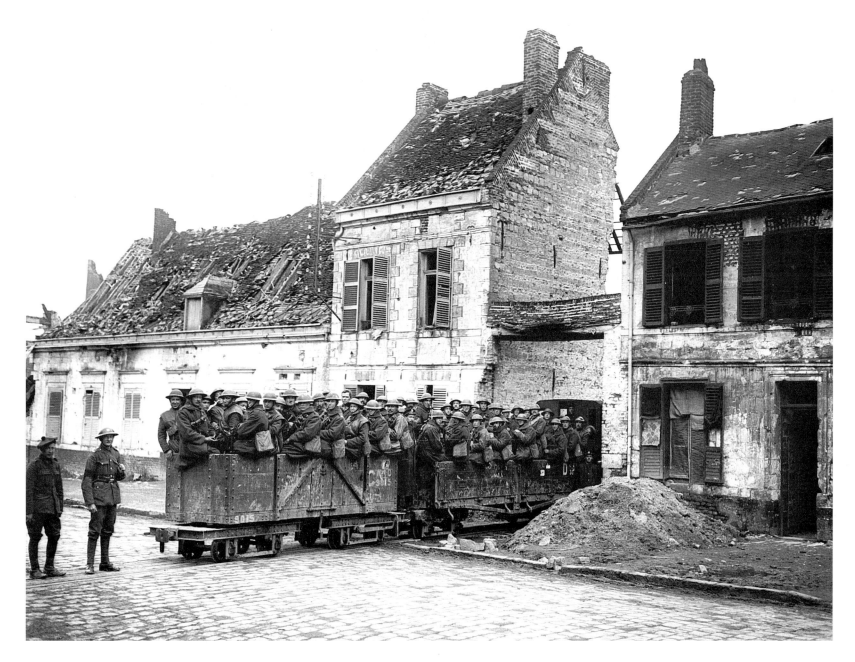

invaluable. The problem was that there simply weren't enough of them. As *The Times'* correspondent in Calcutta, Howard Russell, wrote at the time:

> One is weary of thinking how much blood, disgrace, misery and horror had been saved to us if the rail had been but a little longer here, had been at all there, had been completed in another place. It has been a heavy mileage of neglect for which we have paid dearly.

The railways' potential for help in countering internal unrest continued to be appreciated. At the opening of the New York subway in 1900 the police commissioner rejoiced: 'This subway is going to absolutely preclude the possibility of riots in New York. If a riot should break out at any time now we could clear the road and send out a trainload of a thousand men and have an armed force in Harlem in fifteen minutes.' Twenty years later the Russian revolutionary government used the Tsarist railway network radiating outwards from Moscow with great effect to quash the many rebels who still held out against Communist rule.

Well before 1917 the art of using railways in fighting against external enemies had been fully explored – and their limitations found wanting. Yet they had originally provided a revolutionary response to Napoleon's famous cry: 'Only give me time.' They offered a unique opportunity for his successors to compress time and gain the crucial advantage of surprise in battle. Indeed it was only the railways, with their ability to move seemingly unlimited reinforcements of men and supplies at 32 km (20 miles) every hour, instead of the day required for horse-drawn wagons to cover the same distance, which brought about the fulfilment of the dream of the French revolutionaries, of a nation in arms.

Two years after the Indian Mutiny it was the French who used railways for the first time against an external enemy by rushing troops to Italy in Napoleonic fashion to fight the Emperor of Austria. And only a few years later the use of railways in wartime reached its peak of sophistication in the American Civil War. The Americans had always been alert to their military potential. One of the reasons why the people of Baltimore had promoted the country's first railway in 1828 was to bring in reinforcements at short notice should the wicked British attempt to repeat their success of a mere sixteen years earlier in capturing the city from the sea.

In fact the Civil War was the first 'railway war', in which all the railways' importance was assumed by all sides and all their advantages and limitations were fully explored. Indeed, thanks to the improvements carried out with Federal funds, the railways in the North ended the war in far better shape than before, with far stronger track and a far more unified gauge. By contrast the Confederate railroads were in a terrible state by the end of the war. When General Porter captured one of them in 1865 he observed that its 'undulations were so striking that a train moving along it looked in the distance like a fly crawling across a corrugated washboard.'

The war symbolized the North's industrial supremacy, which gradually imposed a grip on the Confederacy so tight that not even the brilliance of its generals could break. The alliance between the Union's politicians and generals and the railway managers pressed into their service was the first time a chain had been formed which was to be recreated whenever the United States was deemed to be in danger again, whether from Fascism or Communism. It was the prototype of what was to become known as the 'military industrial complex'.

The North had relied on railways from the very start. When Washington was under attack just after the outbreak of war, the Unionist general, Ben Butler, could not pass through Baltimore, where the bridges had been burnt. He shipped his troops down the Potomac river to Annapolis, where he commandeered a rusty old locomotive and called for volunteers to repair it. Immediately a private stepped up with the claim, 'That engine was built in our shops, I guess I can fit her up and run her.' He could and did, and Butler arrived in time to save the capital.

The northerners' skills were not only technical, they were also managerial. The Unionists naturally enlisted the talents of men like Thomas Scott, boss of the fabled Pennsylvania Railroad and Assistant Secretary of War. He set up a separate railroad corps within the army, led by Daniel C. McCallum, a man of many and varied talents (he was a poet and architect as well as a successful railroad executive).

McCallum was lucky: he was given complete authority over the rails. By contrast the Confederates were fighting against central control so they were psychologically and politically unable to impose the same grip as the Unionists on their railways – whose

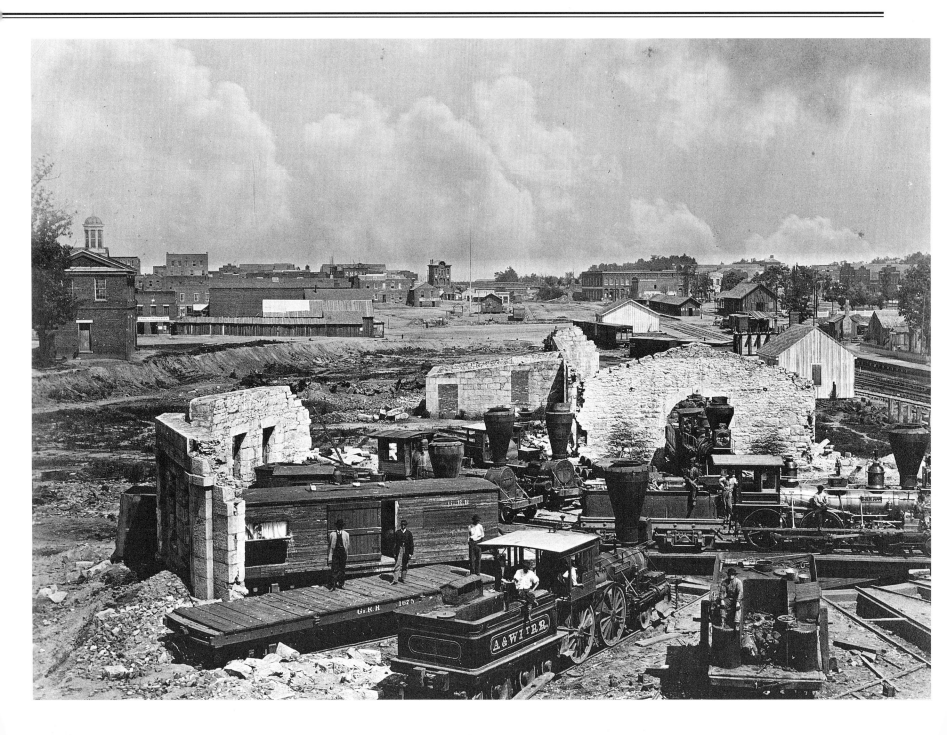

bosses saw their first duty as being to their shareholders, even in wartime. At the same time the Civil War provided the first demonstration of a fact which was to become even clearer in later conflicts – that only railwaymen, not generals, could organize the scale of transport facilities required by the military.

But even the talented McCallum was outshone by two geniusses: a general, William Tecsumah Sherman, and an engineer, Herman Haupt. Haupt was a brilliant organizer – the system of ambulance trains he devised was said to be worth an extra 100,000 men to the Union Army: but his greatest genius lay in his capacity to build and repair track, and above all bridges. By the end of the war he and McCallum had organized the building of more than 2000 miles (3200 km) of military railroads. But he is best known for inspiring President Lincoln's oft-quoted remark: 'That man Haupt has built a bridge across Potomac Creek ... over which loaded trains are running every hour, and, upon my word, gentlemen, there is nothing in it but beanpoles and cornstalks.'

Operationally, the war's most distinguished 'railway general', whose understanding of their strategic potential has never been surpassed, was William Sherman. In the summer of 1864, Sherman reached Atlanta by using railroads to sweep round the southern flanks of the Appalachian mountains, in his revolutionary 'indirect approach.' Sherman had identified Atlanta as the nodal point of transport and industry in the mid-south and knew that if he could eliminate it the Confederacy would be split. His tactic, original at the time but endlessly analysed and copied over the following century, was to keep hooking round the city and thus cutting the enemy's supply lines, ensuring that the final assault would be on a weakened and bewildered force. His nominal superior, General Ulysses S. Grant, also showed considerable understanding of the use of railroads by ensuring that Sherman's opponent, Robert E. Lee, couldn't use them to send reinforcements. But Sherman was sophisticated enough not to cling to railroads, vulnerable to sabotage, when they ran through hostile territory where he preferred to rely on water-borne transport.

European generals, particularly the General Staff of the Prussian army, were certainly not going to learn from the Americans, whom they regarded as amateurs in the art of

Opposite *A classic image of the American Civil War: Sherman's occupation of the demolished engine roundhouse in Atlanta, Georgia.*

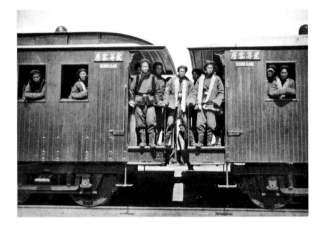

The army of the Manchus travelling in comfort on the Manchurian section of the Trans-Siberian, to try (unsuccessfully) to quash the 1911 revolution.

Opposite *Seventy years later, the same section of the line is being used to transport conscripts, naturally shabby, as befits members of what the Chinese call the 'People's Liberation Army'.*

war. But Helmut von Moltke, the genius of the Prussian army, was a railway enthusiast who had first demonstrated their military potential in 1866, when Germany still contained numerous separate railway systems belonging to the individual states. He was able to use five separate systems to rush 285,000 men to the Austrian border (the better-organized Austrian railways only had one track so couldn't move so fast).

Although the Franco-Prussian war four years later is always held up as an example of the value of railways, and of the German superiority in using them, in fact the French had a better-organized railway system than the Prussians. The Prussian victory was due to political and non-railway factors (notably that Napoleon III had scattered his army all over France to eliminate any possibility of a military coup).

Indeed, although the railways helped the Prussians enormously in their initial victories, they soon showed their limitations. They couldn't deliver enough provisions to supply the troops occupying Northern France, and the tracks proved as vulnerable to sabotage in hostile territory as Sherman had anticipated.

Even more effective, especially in a barren and hostile environment, were lightly-armed cavalry. In the Boer War the British had to station troops in innumerable blockhouses along thousands of miles of railway, most importantly on the line from Cape Town to the front, to repulse attacks from a relatively small number of Boer cavalrymen. But the most glamorous example of the vulnerability of isolated railway lines occurred in the First World War when Colonel T. E. Lawrence ('of Arabia') cut the railway line which was the Turks' only means of supplying their far-flung troops in the desert. As a result 25,000 troops were pinned in blockhouses along the line, and the garrison at Medina, the key to Mecca, was completely helpless.

Railways could not necessarily prove the answer to a general's prayer. For a start their capacity was limited: in their war against Japan in 1904–1906 the Russians found it impossible to supply their troops in the Far East along the single-track, still uncompleted Trans-Siberian Railway – it did not help that a number of Grand Dukes commandeered trains for their personal use. Nevertheless the war did a great deal to reduce the line's fatal limitations. When war broke out the Russians expected to operate only three pairs of trains every day, but loops were built, track and bridges strengthened in key places

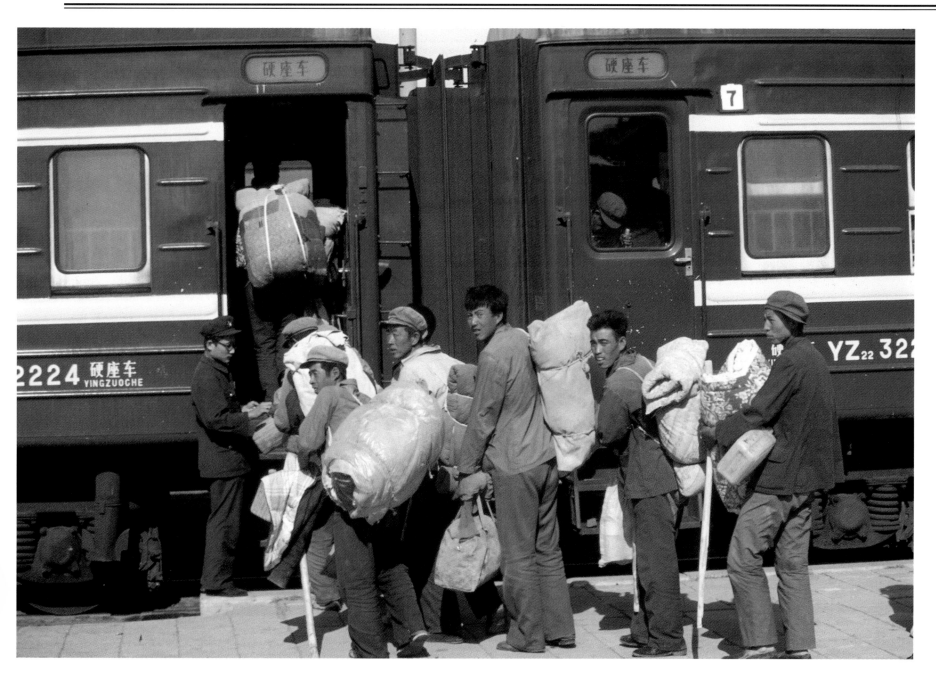

and proper schedules introduced for the first time. By the end of the war it could handle sixteen pairs of trains a day.

By 1914, it seemed, planning, involving the movement of masses of troops, had become a substitute for thought, so far as the general staffs of the Great Powers were concerned. In the railway age the movement of troops and supplies had to be planned well in advance, and emergency timetables could not be improvized on the spot. This had been possible in the previous era of horse transport and was again possible once masses of trucks were available.

The inflexibility of the rail-borne war machine built on the back of the railways' unique capacity to mobilize armies has been blamed for the outbreak of war. Many historians believed that the German plans could not have been changed, the invasion of Belgium could not have been stopped, after the Kaiser had changed his mind. In fact the error was human: it was the fault of the Chief of the German general staff, the 'great' von Moltke's nephew, who could have countermanded the order if he had not been living in the shadow of his uncle's martial reputation.

But in any case the railways were already dictating the nature of the war, a type of warfare where operations were inevitably fairly rigid until the internal combustion engine restored flexibility to the military menu. But the events of 1914 rubbed in the truth of the words of Colonel G. F. R. Henderson, in *The Science of War* published six years earlier: 'Railways in war are good servants but bad masters.'

Railways were soon reduced to acting merely as – albeit essential – supply lines, but in August 1914 two major battles had been won by generals who understood their strategic value. Marshal Joffre, himself a former railwayman, used railways in a masterful move of troops from his right to his left flank, and thus saved the French army in the Battle of the Marne. And when the Russians invaded East Prussia the Germans could rush two army corps to their theatened frontier in time for them to win the crucial battle of Tannenberg.

In the west the war soon settled down to an appalling battle of attrition and the railways came to fulfil another vital role, not tactical, let alone strategic, but logistic. The use of automatic weapons which so drastically changed the balance of advantage between

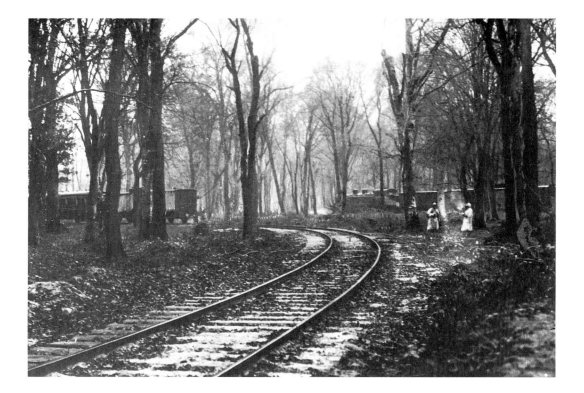

Dawn on 11 November 1918; five hours before the Armistice was signed in the coach on the left of the picture.

the defenders and the attackers would not have been possible without the vastly increased supplies of ammunition which only the railways had the capacity to carry.

But more memorable for the survivors were the troop trains. The nonagenarian Frederick Hodges, then an infantry corporal, remembers how they were by no means luxurious: 'Painted on them in white letters was *hommes 40 chevaux 8* – and we knew what that meant and there was straw of a sort – very dirty – for us to sit down and lie on, but we were too active to sit down – we wanted to know what was going on. Some of us climbed up onto the roof to travel like they do in Asia, and the others were firing their rifles, 'cause we'd never been given possession of ammunition before. [The trains were] very long and they never went at any speed, they sometimes stopped for unknown reasons, we even got out and walked by the side of them sometimes.'

They remained a crucial symbol and it seemed natural for the victorious allies to use a railway carriage (number 2419, borrowed for the purpose from the Orient Express) as the scene for the signing of the Armistice in November 1918. It was equally natural for

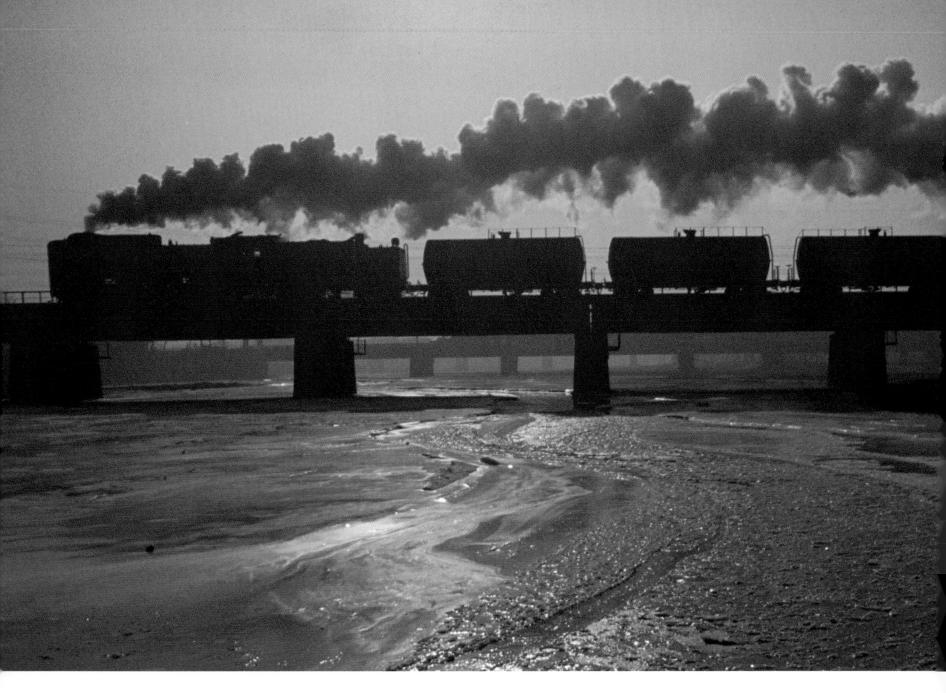

Railways remained crucial for supply purposes in wartime. Even all-conquering tanks were helpless without the sort of oil train pictured here in Manchuria.

88

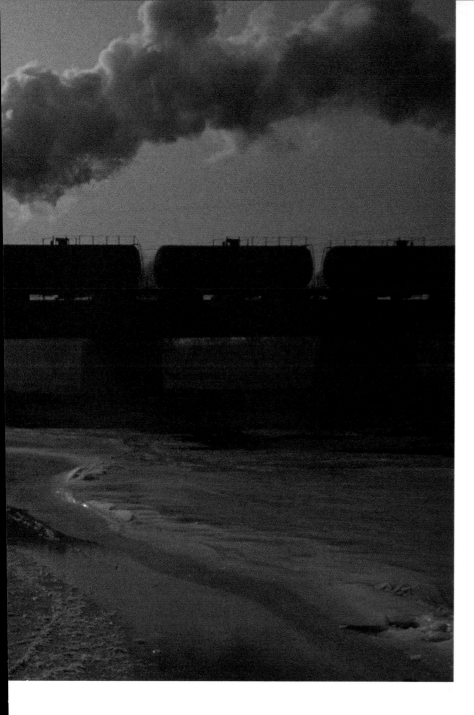

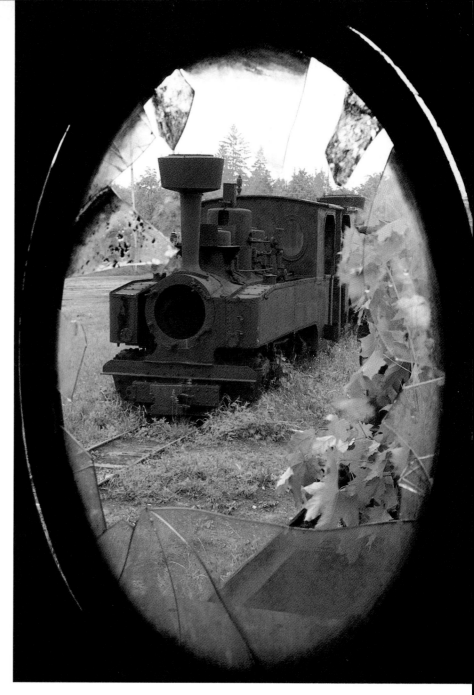

Graveyard of a loyal servant. A former 'Feldbahn' German military engine at rest after being used on a forest railway in Poland.

Hitler to use the same carriage to receive the French surrender in June 1940, and equally appropriate that the SS blew it up four years later to prevent a third symbolic event.

In the popular imagination, the Second World War was symbolized less by carriages like number 2419 than by aircraft and tanks. But railways remained the essential sinews of the war effort for all the participants. Trucks could never supply the increasing quantity of supplies required by a modern army. Obviously the longer the distances involved the more essential they were, a point of special importance on the Russian front. But at first the Germans did not realize their importance. Hitler had assumed that the war would be over after the initial blitzkrieg and, because of the Germans' reliance on autobahns, they had fewer locomotives at their disposal than they had had in 1914.

Worse, even after their appalling initial defeats the Russians continued to resist and tore up the tracks before they retreated. By the winter of 1941 the assumptions that the war would be won before Christmas, and that it could be fought using primarily road transport had both already proved false. In the west the blitzkrieg had worked – and there were adequate roads to carry the supplies required. In Russia neither was true.

The Russians rubbed in the importance of railways when they used the Trans-Siberian to move the whole of their heavy industry away from the invading Germans from the Ukraine and western Russia to safety east of the Urals – one factory alone, the steel works from Zaporozhstal, required 8000 railway wagons. Strategically the Russians could use the Trans-Siberian to bring their 'Winter Army' thousands of miles west from Manchuria to save Moscow from the Germans in the winter of 1941. Later in the war only their railways could supply enough ammunition for the 40,000 guns with which they pounded the German forces.

Although most of the supplies brought by the Allies arrived by sea via Murmansk, another railway line, the one built by Reza Shah across Persia in the 1920s, proved crucial – especially after the Americans took over its operation from the British who had moved only 200,000 tons of supplies along the tracks during the whole of 1942. Then 4000 troops from the Transport Corps formed in 1942 arrived and within a short time they were transporting 180,000 tons a month over the same route.

Throughout the war the Germans suffered from what has been called 'mixed media' forms of transport. They relied more than anyone realized at the time on horses, which, unlike motor transport, could move in the depths of the Russian winter, when the roads were seas of frozen mud. But the Germans then grasped the crucial need for the railways. Hitler centralized control in Berlin and placed the whole thing in the hands of the railwaymen, who had the power to overrule the army – a fruitful source of conflict when officers were battling to move train-loads of wounded troops back to base.

The Germans then had to cope with the uncomfortable fact that the gauge of the tracks east of Brest Litovsk in Poland was a few centimetres wider than those in the rest of Europe, and that, partly because of the efficacy of Russian scorched earth tactics, there was an acute shortage of locomotives. The first problem was partly solved by massive 'regauging' of Russian lines down to the German standard, with the help of Russian prisoners of war (who were paid half a kilo of salt a day). But the Germans' insistence on setting standards, that so many kilometres had to be regauged every day, meant that points and intersections were neglected, so the regauged lines could not be fully exploited. And since not all the sabotaged signalling equipment was replaced the trains could travel only by day, and then had to rely on watching for trains in front.

The locomotive problem was solved through the *Kriegslocomotiv*, a crash programme of building specially designed freight engines, with closed cabs and bunks for the crew, using thousands of suppliers from all over the Reich. The British and Americans went in for similar programmes with their 'Austerity' and 'Macarthur' engines respectively. The German programme was indeed successful: within three years they had built 7000 engines, each of which took only 8000 man-hours to build, as against 22,000 for a peacetime locomotive.

Bombing proved less effective than ground sabotage in wrecking railway networks – although for a long time 'Bomber' Harris of Bomber Command refused to countenance attacks on targets as specific as railway stations or marshalling yards. This was an admission of his bombers' inadequate capacity to hit specific targets. As Roland Beamont, an ace pilot explains: 'we had very little in the way of navigational aids in those days and unless the marshalling yards were in a large city with fairly prominent landmarks around it, it was a very difficult thing to pick 'em up, very ... extremely difficult.'

Typically, the Bielefeld viaduct, a vital link between Hamm in the Ruhr and Hanover, remained undamaged until March 1945, when one of Barnes Wallis's bouncing bombs, a 10-tonne (22,000-lb) monster named 'Grand Slam', finally destroyed it – although by then the Germans had built a well-camouflaged alternative route round the side of the valley which the viaduct had spanned. After two years of bombardment the landscape round it resembled the craters of the moon, yet the railway was still running.

By 1944 bomb sights had greatly improved and the bombers showed their paces above all in France, where the Allies were unhappy about bombing towns, a reticence which, ironically, made their bombing tactics far more effective militarily than the saturation bombing in Germany.

As Beamont explains: 'If you dropped bombs on the tracks they were rather difficult to hit and they were easy to repair ... if you attacked the tracks with guns you weren't going to do any harm, your shells would bounce off the tracks but if you went for the engine you could knock the engine out and that stopped the train.'

But Beamont and his colleagues found that the Typhoon and Tempest fighter-bombers developed in 1943–44 were ideal for the purpose: 'the combination of accurate gun aiming, heavy armament and high speed made it a very good aeroplane for ground attack and for attacking locomotives.' To record their successes and improve the morale of the ground crews, pilots like Beamont painted locomotives on the sides of their planes to record successful attacks. They were especially valuable before and after D-Day when the Germans were unable to move Panzer divisions to the front: thanks to the bombardments a crucial SS armoured division was held up for two weeks. The Germans' effort was also undermined by the sabotage efforts of the French railway workers, the deservedly much-praised *cheminots*. They were in a good position to help, able to move and to carry messages without attracting suspicion (messages were regularly carried between Paris and Vichy, the seat of the collaborationist government, in the tender of the engine hauling the Prime Minister, Pierre Laval).

By 1943 the *cheminots* were able to resist more openly, at first by stealth – they would let waybills get lost, spares would be misplaced, bulbs were removed to hamper work at night, coal would be thrown onto the track so that the trains would run out of fuel.

Opposite *An artist's view of the Blitz: Norman Wilkinson's dramatic image of an attack on the key marshalling yards at Willesden in North West London at the end of 1940.*

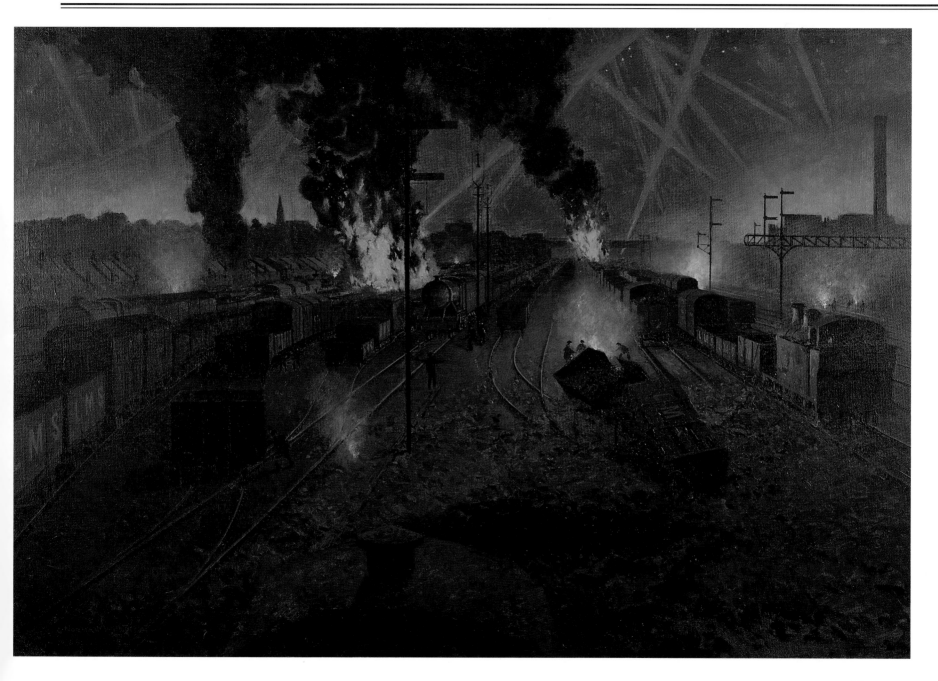

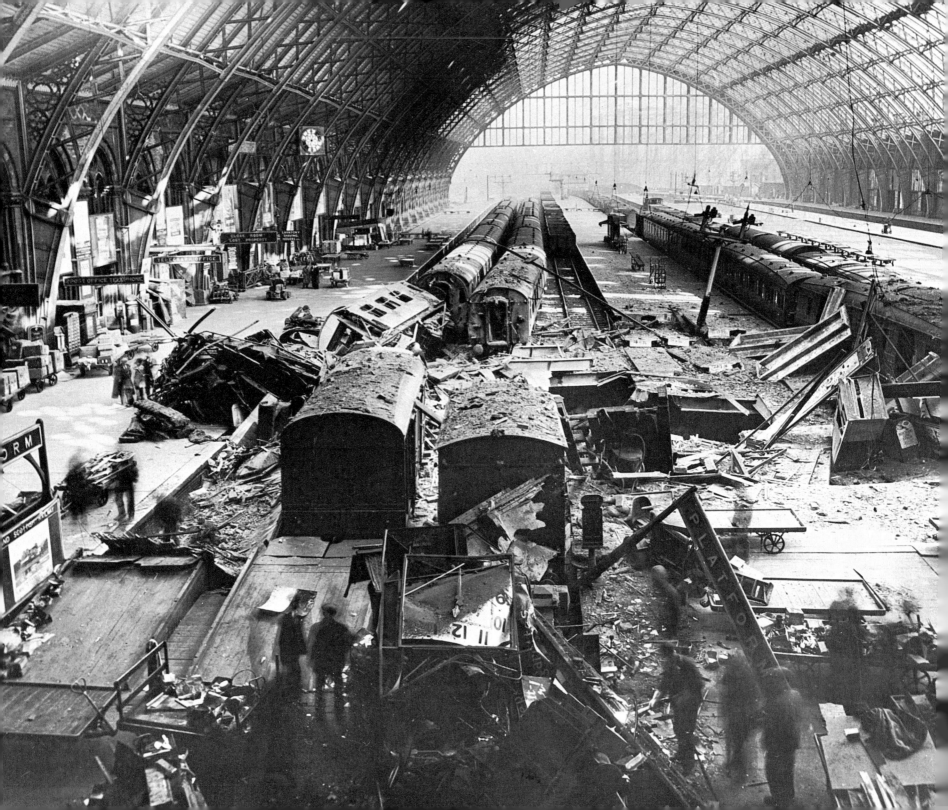

Then came outright sabotage: 6000 trains were derailed – and in retaliation 800 railwaymen were shot and another 1150 sent to concentration camps. Indeed the combination of precision bombing and the *cheminots'* efforts after D-Day merely emphasized the point first appreciated by General Sherman eighty years earlier, that railways were both inflexible and vulnerable in wartime.

Cruelly, by the end of the war, the only trains that seemed to move with any regularity inside the rapidly-shrinking Reich were those carrying thousands of Jews to the extermination camps, the death trains which continued to enjoy an absolute priority over other rail-borne traffic until the very end of the war. Indeed only the existence of a comprehensive railway system enabled the Nazis to transport as many Jews as they did from all over Europe to a handful of camps. Railways played such a crucial role within the Holocaust that at his trial Adolf Eichmann claimed that he was merely a transport officer.

Stalin had always understood the importance of railways – in his days as a youthful revolutionary he had filled the party's coffers with the proceeds from hijacking a train. And in 1945 he arrived at Potsdam in his own train running straight through from Moscow to Berlin after German prisoners of war had regauged the tracks from Brest-Litovsk. According to one survivor, Manfred Mauthner, 'Many people escaped but the Russians would just take new people off the streets to have the right number of workers. We were fed with dog food and sometimes with soup.'

As a result of his experiences Stalin naturally assumed that when he blocked the railway lines connecting Berlin with the West in 1948 the city would be starved into submission. But the Berlin airlift proved him wrong, and emphasized that, militarily at least, the railways' day was done.

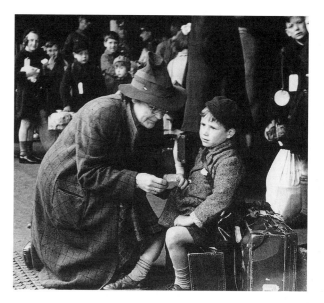

One of a hundred thousand tiny tragic figures thrown up by the mass evacuation of children from London in 1939.

Opposite The quirks of bomb damage: the Great Shed at St Pancras in London is relatively unscathed despite the devastated platforms.

5   *Imperial Power*

The first imperialism introduced by the railway was technical and linguistic: the British who developed the techniques of steam locomotion and the gauge their trains ran on, and whose locomotives were exported and imitated throughout the world left their mark. Although most countries took pride in developing their own rolling stock as soon as possible one legacy remained: the terms used to describe the phenomena associated with the railways. Words like 'train', 'locomotive' and 'station' became common to most languages – although the French and the Germans had sufficient sense of their own cultural identity to coin many of their own terms.

The imperialism which so dominated the nineteenth century was itself profoundly influenced by the railways. Railways created colonies like Kenya, and enabled small groups of men, like the British in India, to rule a continent. On an even larger scale the Trans-Siberian Railway created Siberia and colonized it with millions of Russians. And because the lines required such great amounts of capital they could not be financed by many of the countries in what we would now call the Third World. So they, and the finance they required, became the first symbol of 'indirect imperialism', the dominance of supposedly independent countries by international financial institutions. Today, although direct imperialism is a thing of the past, the arguments over the political and financial relationships involved in indirect imperialism continue to embitter the dialogue between the developed and underdeveloped worlds.

Indeed railways were generally built for the convenience of the imperial conqueror, and its need to defend itself either against the natives or against threat from a rival power. The result was a patchwork of development, since the authorities at home were

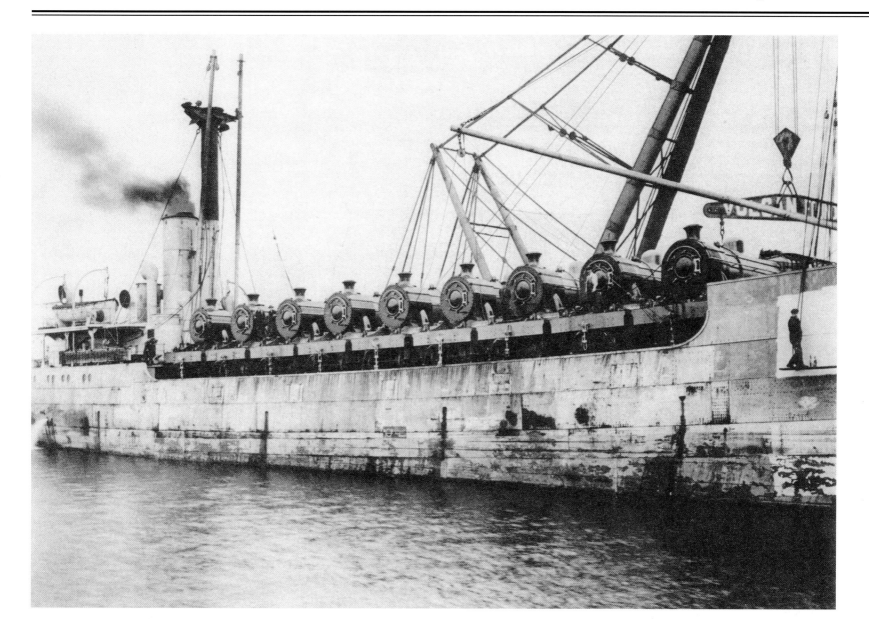

Imperialism in action: locomotives destined for India being shipped from Birkenhead in 1930.

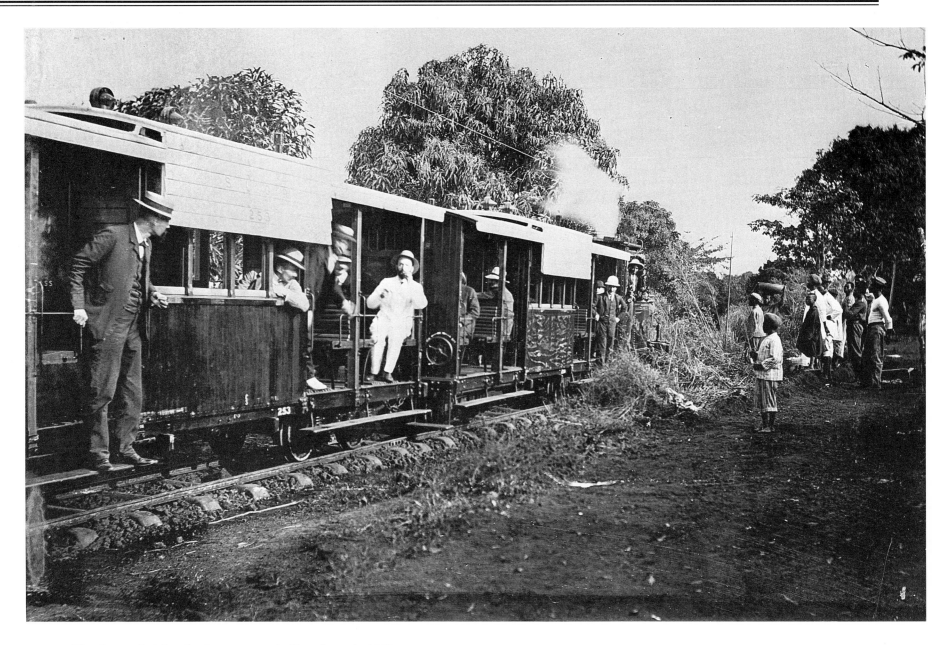

The charm of a leisurely trip up-country in Sierra Leone in 1903.

reluctant to finance railways in normal times, and generally granted the funds only when there was (or seemed to be) some unacceptable threat from a rival. The classic case is the so-called 'Lunatic Line' from Mombasa on the Indian Ocean to the shores of Lake Victoria in what became Uganda. It was promoted for the usual mixed reasons: to bring Christianity (and thus, by implication, civilization) to the benighted natives, and to forestall the ambitions of the Germans, who had already occupied what became Tanganyika. Despite the hostility shown by many British politicians – hence its derisory nickname – the line created Kenya and its capital, Nairobi, originally merely the station at the point where the line started to climb into the hills.

If railways outside already developed countries were to be self-financing, they had to depend on some mineral resource or cash crop. Except in China and India there was no possible profit from linking existing towns and cities. The results were often rather odd. By 1910 the French had extended their railway north from Hanoi in what was then French Indo-China to Kunming in southern China for vaguely imperialist reasons – and to get at the province's riches in silk, minerals, leather, furs and precious stones. So for decades it was easier to go from Shanghai to Kunming via Hanoi, hundreds of miles to the south than directly overland.

The mixture of motives on the part of the imperialists was matched by a similar ambivalence on the part of nationalists outside Europe fighting to be free from colonialism: railways were symbols of modernity, and thus a good thing; but at the same time they were being imposed as part of an alien culture, and thus a bad thing. It made matters worse that railways epitomized the inferiority imposed on the natives. Few natives travelled first class on Indian railways, and in Indo-China in the 1930s the French operated special luxury railcars reserved for their exclusive use.

As so often, India provides a classic example of all the effects and the contradictions involved in imperial history. To the emerging nationalist movement railways were at once a symbol of imperial rule and an essential element in uniting the country sufficiently to enable a nationalist party to fight effectively against it. Railways became a symbol of the Raj, of colonial exploitation and systematic racism but, equally, they contributed greatly to the economic development of the subcontinent.

Right *India old and new: a train bound for Agra passes a group of women washing in the Yamuna River. Note the length of the bridge, designed to cope with a river in flood.*

Below *The dining-car attendants on an Indian train have to be agile because the door between the dining-car and First Class carriages is locked for security reasons.*

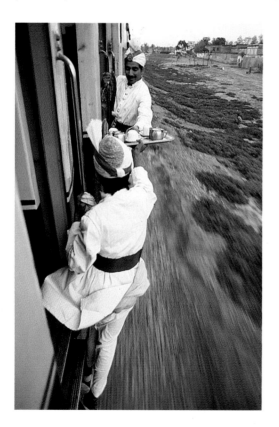

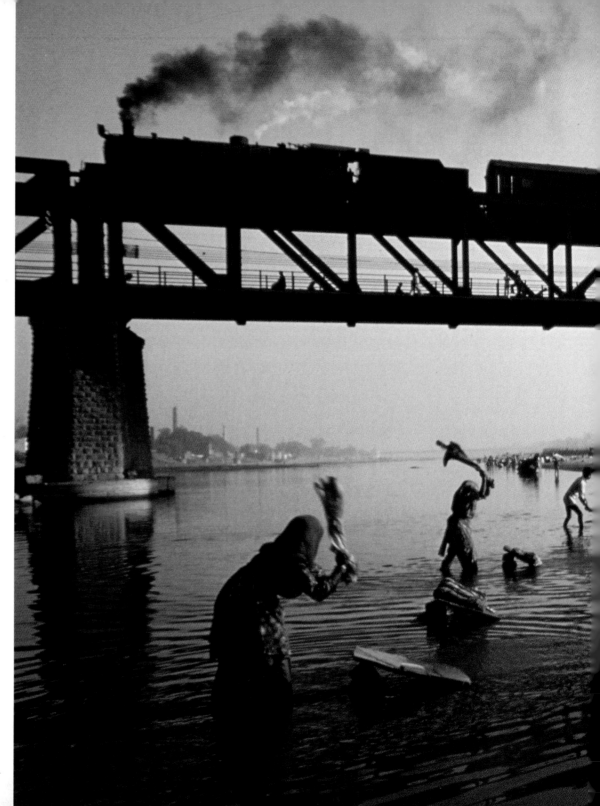

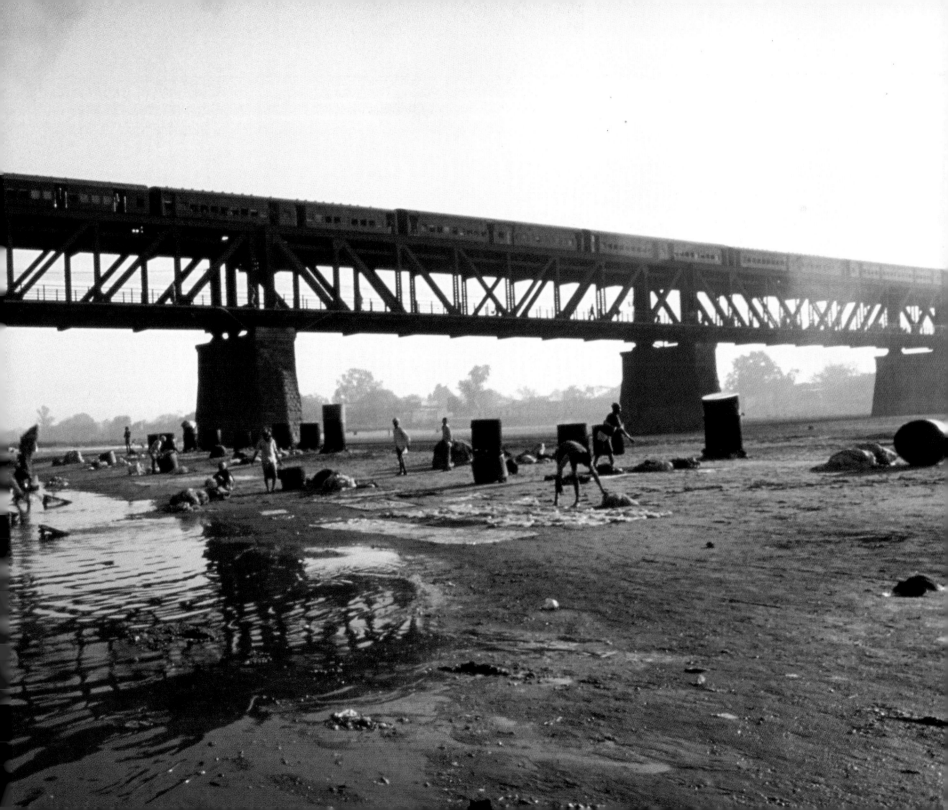

As a primary symbol of the modernization and imperial control the British brought in their train, the first few lines were a prime target for the mutineers in 1857 trying to return to earlier days and ways. For railways were perceived, and not only by the Indians, as embodying a fundamental threat to their spiritual and social existence; indeed the British naively hoped they would carry missionaries the length and breadth of the country. In Edward Davidson's *The Railways of India*, published as early as 1868:

> The evangelists … implied that the benefits of western civilization were inseparable from worship of the western god: if the Indians wanted railways they would have to have God as well. Thus to fervent Hindus the railways were associated with an attack on their souls. It was not just the question of gods: the very nature of the railway, demanding punctuality and exactitude, breaking down caste, was also alien.

As we saw in Chapter 4, the Mutiny was a decisive factor in speeding up the development of a rail system in the subcontinent. But, as usual with such imperial ventures, a mixture of motives was at work: more effective control of the country, economic development, private profit, and as a defence against a perceived Russian menace (as late as 1987 the blockhouses built a century earlier to protect the stations on the lines to the Afghan border housed racks of ancient Lee-Enfield rifles). The muddle of motives was reflected in the different methods employed to finance new lines.

Initially there was great enthusiasm among secular-minded Indians for railways, but it soon became clear that they were to have no say in financing or running them. For railways were closely linked with the Raj. Originally financed by government money, the mixed financial pattern which eventually emerged – not as a deliberate policy but the result of the imperial power's combination of meanness, vacillation and desire for control – provided the imperial government with a large part of its revenues from the lines under state control, as well as a network of privately-owned lines which could be used by the Raj to prevent any repetition of unrest. Following the Mutiny it was decreed that no line should be built which would not bear the weight of an Armstrong gun. Davidson quoted an official view that 'the Empire is safer with 50,000 troops and the rail than it could be with double that and no rail.'

The system inevitably reflected, indeed encouraged, the strict racial segregation which characterized India under British rule for over half a century after the Mutiny. The pattern was three-fold, with the natives doing the hard work, a smaller group of (often expatriate) white supervisors and Anglo-Indians in between. Socially, the Anglo-Indians were stranded and thus acted as a reliable buffer between the natives and their white rulers. For they were at home only in their recognized role as the non-commissioned officers in the million-strong army of steam, in which they furnished the clerks, the foremen. They were loyal to their superiors and could be relied on to keep control over their 'native' inferiors – during the great railway strike of 1922, for instance, they sided with their masters.

The situation was naturally perceived by later generations of Indian nationalists as an imperialist plot, and not always without reason. The great Indian economist, Romesh Chandra Dutt, was among many Indians who considered expenditure on railways as wasteful compared with money spent on roads or even canals. Gandhi was, bluntly, two-faced on the subject. His missionary efforts depended on his ability to travel, mostly by train, throughout India. Yet at the same time he could attack railways for exacerbating famines (which was a blatant lie, they were crucial in reducing their effect). He also believed that good travelled at a snail's pace and that industrialization, of which the railways were a prime symbol, was evil, so that railways 'drew man further away from his maker', and 'accentuated the evil nature of man ... thus enabling ... bad men to fulfil their evil designs with greater rapidity.'

The two observers who best understood the impact of railways on India and their relationship with British rule were that curious pair Karl Marx and Rudyard Kipling – whose first books were published as part of the Indian Railway Library launched by a local publisher, A. H. Wheeler & Co. Kipling's magic story, *The Bridge Builders*, tells of the power of the monsoon and of the Ganges, of the Hindu gods' displeasure at the taming of so mighty a river by a railway bridge and of the engineer-designer's shame at the possibility of it cracking under the strain (he does, it doesn't). For his part Marx, in *Future Results of the British Rule in India*, saw that 'England has to fulfil a double mission in India: one destructive, and the other regenerative – the annihilation of old Asiatic society, and the laying of the material foundations of western society in India.'

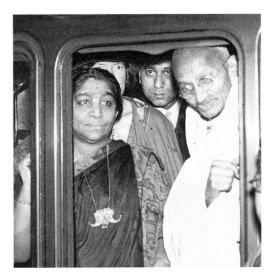

Mahatma Gandhi never explained the paradox: he travelled by train to help him spread his message that industrialization (i.e. railways) was evil.

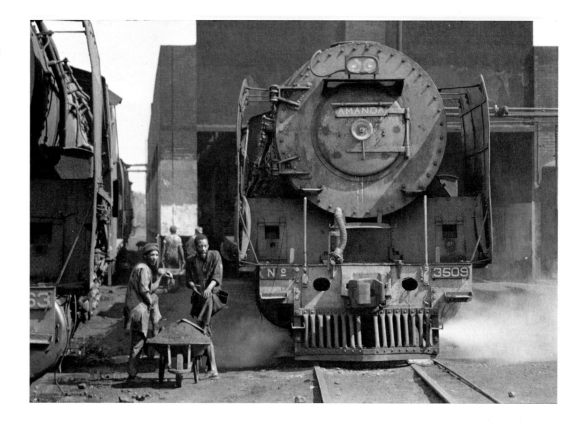

A train with the improbable name of Amanda, at De Aar, a major railway junction north of Cape Town.

Indian railways were also a crucial symbol of the Great Game played out in the Himalayas between Britain and Russia, a 'Game' resembling Grandmother's Footsteps, albeit one played on an imperial scale. By 1885 the Russians had laid tracks as far as Merv, well on the way from the Caspian Sea to the Afghan border, and pushed on through appalling desert conditions with a line whose use was primarily strategic. The British in India responded with an extension to the Kandahar State railway which, with typical British love of secrecy, was called the 'Henrai Road improvement scheme.' Later on, the Sind Peshia state railway was extended to Chaman, within 400 yds (365 metres) of the Afghan frontier, complete with stores ready to lay the 52 miles (83 km) within Afghanistan to Kandahar.

The Great Game was but one instance of a world-wide pattern in which the great powers used railways as weapons against each other. This applied even to railways in Europe itself. Before the Swiss took control of their own destiny their country could be classed in historical terms as a sector where the burgeoning imperialism of France and Germany clashed – well before the imperial powers used railways, real or planned, as a weapon in the Middle East, Morocco, the Balkans, and, more especially, in Africa, where imperial rivalry left a permanent legacy. In 1988 the Economist Intelligence Unit wrote: 'A century ago both Kruger and Rhodes observed that control of Southern Africa lay in control of the rail network. To a remarkable extent that statement remains true today.'

Indeed railways throughout Africa remain a hotchpotch of lines, rather than proper systems, because they were built patchily, either as a result of economic opportunism – like the lines to the mines of Zambia and the Belgian Congo – or because of attempts by the British, the French or the Germans to second-guess their rivals and establish control over a region through the building of a railway line.

Every imperial country dreamed its own dreams, to use railways either to preserve or extend their dominions. The Tsar's imperial ambitions (and fears) played a large part in the long-discussed decision to build a railway across Siberia to the Pacific, and two other crumbling empires also saw railways as a means of preserving their sway. The first major line in the Austro-Hungarian Empire was designed to link the capital, Vienna, with Trieste, the Empire's major seaport, and the Ottoman Emperors used railways, mostly built with foreign money, to tighten their grip on their far-flung empire, from the Balkans to the southern tip of Arabia.

The Germans were even more ambitious. Like the other imperial powers in Africa they had built a number of railways in such colonies as Tanganyika and South West Africa, but funds for them were granted grudgingly by the Reichstag – as reluctantly as by their fellow-legislators in Britain and France. But the German people were wholeheartedly behind their greatest imperial dream, a railway from Berlin to Baghdad, which would give them control of the whole Near and Middle East, most obviously the newly-discovered oilfields in Iraq. For the Germans (and for the British) the race for control was between the British fleet and German railway engineers.

The race was not as one-sided as it appears in hindsight. German engineers – notably Wilhelm von Pressel – had been deeply involved in building the railways throughout the Ottoman Empire, and Meissner Pasha had been responsible for most of the Hejaz railway from Damascus to Mecca – although he was replaced by a Muslim for the last few hundred miles since no infidel could be allowed near the Holy City. The project was deemed so important that work continued right through the First World War, in which the Turks were allies of the Germans, and by the time of the Armistice the line was open as far as Aleppo in Eastern Syria. But without the imperial impulse it was never completed – it was never going to be sufficiently profitable to attract enough ordinary capitalist finance.

The British, the greatest imperialists of them all, proved equally hard-headed in their great imperial dream, a British-controlled route from the Cape of Good Hope to Cairo. It was diverted hundreds of miles from its most direct route by one of the greatest of all imperialists, Cecil Rhodes, to help develop what became the copper belt in Northern Rhodesia. And it was the Marquess of Salisbury, considered Britain's most imperial-minded Prime Minister, who finally scuppered the whole idea when, in one of the imperial carve-ups so typical of the day and age, he allowed the Germans sway over Tanganyika as far west as the Belgian Congo, thus leaving no room for a British-controlled railway to pass.

The British abandoned the Cape-to-Cairo route largely because it was simply too megalomaniac a notion for so practical a people. By contrast the French continued to plan an apparently much more far-fetched idea, a railway right across the Sahara. For half a century this mad idea was supported by a number of interested parties: by generals anxious to extend France's sway east into the Sudan – especially after a famous incident at Fashoda in the South of Sudan, in 1898, when the British repelled French interlopers; and by more practical advocates, anxious to provide France with the means of importing tropical produce from West Africa far more quickly than was otherwise possible – they were undeterred by the mundane fact that a combination of local railways, river transport and steamships was perfectly adequate for the job. As late as 1943 the Vichy government actually started to build the first stretch south from Algeria, as if to emphasize that the German-dominated France they represented was still entitled to its imperial dreams.

Once the Japanese had become an imperial power, they too went in for some suitably imperial railway-building, first through Manchuria. They also indulged in some imperial day-dreaming, planning a tunnel from Southern Japan to the southern tip of Korea, then part of the Japanese empire. They even bought and reserved a strip of land south from Tokyo for the purpose. However ridiculous this seemed at the time, it eventually served a practical purpose, since after the Second World War it was used for the first specially built high-speed line in the world, the Shinkansen between Tokyo and Osaka.

But dream lines were not confined to imperial powers, or indeed to politicians. The Transcontinental railroad across the United States owed its existence to a series of dreamers, culminating in an engineer, who was called 'Crazy Judah' because of his dogged efforts, first in surveying possible routes through the Rockies and the Sierras and then his passionate advocacy of his cause in such unpromising milieux as Wall Street.

The great heroes of the nineteenth century naturally extended their ambitions into grandiose railway schemes. Following his extraordinary success in creating the Suez Canal the French diplomat Ferdinand de Lesseps sent his son Victor to explore the possibility of a railway linking Paris with eastern cities like Bombay and Peking. And only his premature death prevented E. H. Harriman from pressing on with a plan to control a complete round-the-world route, involving his own steamship company across the Pacific, his own railroad through the United States, a newly built line through Manchuria, and running rights over the Trans-Siberian, the sort of 'land-bridge' now being operated by many companies to carry freight between Europe and Japan.

Many other Americans dreamed of a Pan-American railway right down to Patagonia – a dream realized only through the Pan-American highway. Henry Meiggs, builder of most of the spectacular railways from the Pacific over the Andes, wanted to link the Pacific coast with the Atlantic via a railway to the Amazon, and his nephew, C. Minor Keith, planned a line across Central America. But it was left to Adolf Hitler to dream the truly impossible dream. By the end of the war he had elaborated plans for a massive new railway network from Paris in the west through Germany to Istanbul and the Black Sea in the east. This was no ordinary new railway, since the gauge was 5.63 m (18 ft 6 in), over three times the normal one. The trains were to travel on double tracks which enabled them to be of a truly monstrous size – the locomotives were over 7.5 m (25 ft) high and the dining-car resembled that of a grand hotel with ample room for two tables side by side each seating six people.

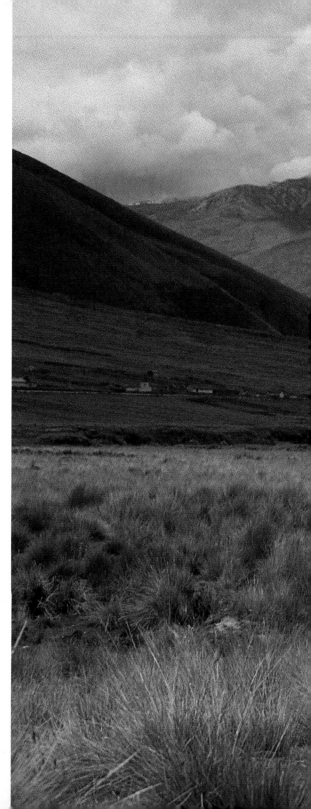

*R*ailways were prime instruments of indirect imperialism, capitalism and exploitation: inevitably, the antics of the men who financed the railways in the developing world turned its inhabitants against the whole idea of capitalism, for they had seen the systematic cheating to which it gave rise, usually ignoring the undeniable benefits which accompanied the financial shenanigans involved.

In China railways became the single most important symbol of foreign exploitation, delaying the development of the country's rail system for two generations. This was not surprising, for it became a natural matter of faith amongst the nationalists fighting the foreign powers which carved their country into 'Spheres of Influence' to treat railways as symbols of imperialist oppression. Occasionally this gave rise to moments of sheer farce. Leopold II of Belgium tried to get concessions in China through nominally independent emissaries from the Free State of the Congo he had created – but the Chinese swiftly spotted the sham, if only because the 'Africans' were stolid white Belgian bourgeois.

As a result the term 'self-built railway' became a key phrase in the nationalists' vocabulary, although when the Chinese did try to build their own they were far less successful than the British, the Belgians, the French and the Americans. This was partly because there were traitors in their own ranks: in Szechuan, a proud, isolated province in the heart of China, attempts to build their own railway in the first decade of the twentieth century were thwarted by the central government in Peking, reckoned to be in league with the foreign oppressors. Although the railway was saved, first by an improbable alliance of patriots and the local mafia and then by the revolution of 1911, construction was at best patchy. The result throughout China was that when Mao and the Communists took over in 1949 only the eastern half of the country had anything like a proper railway network.

In China the imperial powers fought their battles like chess-players, largely ignoring the wishes and needs of the locals. One of the many incidents resulting from this imperialist rivalry was a stand-off between British and Russian troops at Fengtai Junction. Russian troops had advanced along the line from Mukden to Peking, using the Boxer

In the Andes the peasants rely on one of the triumphs of railway engineering.

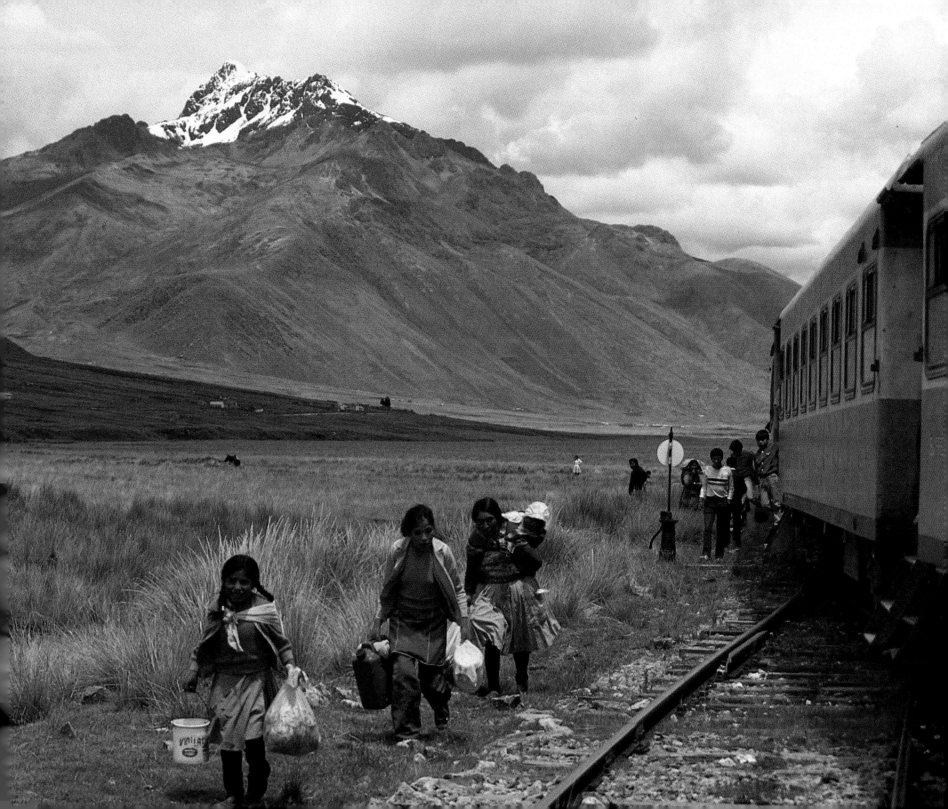

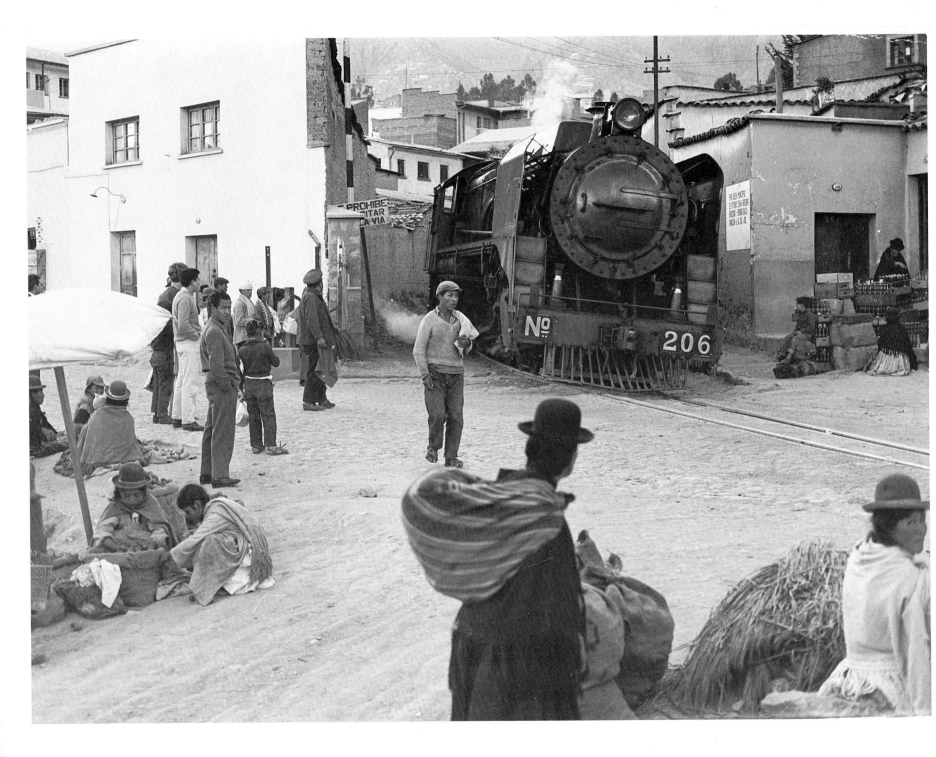

rebellion as an excuse to realize their long-held ambition of linking the Trans-Siberian to the line from Peking to Hangchow in central China and thus dominating the whole of Northern China. British troops successfully faced down the advance with a line of motionless troops levelling their bayonets.

After the Russo-Japanese war the Japanese occupied 700 km (435 miles) of the Chinese Eastern Railway, which the Chinese had previously conceded to Russia. During the First World War the Japanese gained further mileage – although after the Chinese had bought back some of the track the Nanking–Shanghai railway, in particular, was pressed into service, carrying record tonnages to support Chinese troops fighting the Japanese seizure of Southern Manchuria.

*I*n Latin America nationalists were only in favour of railways if they controlled them themselves. And woe betide a leader who allowed the foreigners too much scope. In Mexico much of the blame attached to the regime before the revolution of 1910 was created by President Porfirio Diaz's over-complaisant attitude to foreign capitalists. He was unlucky (or, radicals would say, typical). Apart from Weetman Pearson, the first Lord Cowdray, who built a railway across Mexico to serve both oceans, most of the investors were pretty shady and did little to advance the cause of foreign investment.

Nevertheless nationalists were inclined to overlook impressive statistics: the production of coffee, for example, jumped twenty times in as many years, reaching 28 million pounds by 1890; and only railways enabled the Mexicans to get to market millions of pounds of oranges which would otherwise have rotted on the ground.

Even where the effects were almost uniformly favourable – as in Argentina where British capital provided the country with a splendid network – the resentment generated by the idea that the railways represented imperialist exploitation festered for generations and the boil was burst by President Perón when he nationalized the railways after the war. The result was only too typical: a corrupt and incompetent state administration designed to place as many supporters as possible on the payroll rather than provide services (they are now being reprivatized).

But the nationalists had a point: they had paid heavily for their railways. The

Opposite *La Paz in Bolivia: where the trains run at 12,500 feet (3810 m).*

111

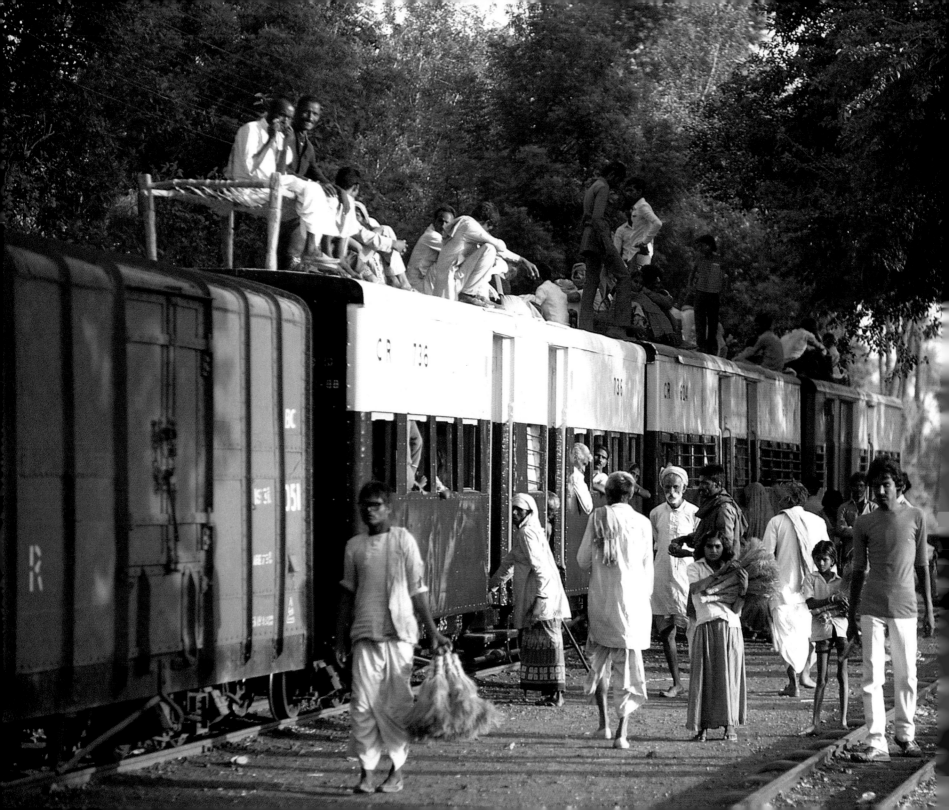

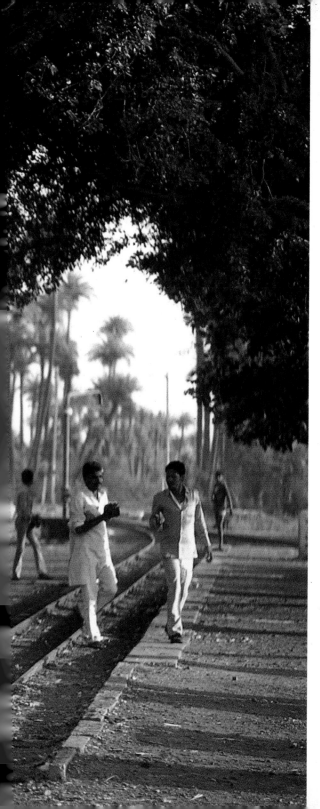

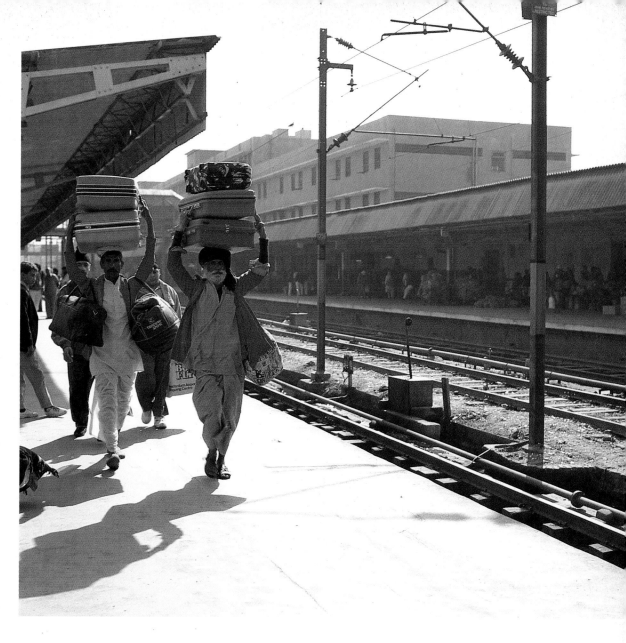

Above *India's eternal contrast: the railway line is electrified, but cheap labour means that passengers at Delhi do not need trolleys for their luggage.*

Left *Once upon a time the Maharaja of Scindia built a little toy railway. But now Bamourgaon station in Madhya Pradesh is part of the state system.*

promoters of new lines made their initial profit by paying the issuing country at a discount to the bonds' face value – typically the Turks received only 60 per cent of the money they had borrowed for their early railways. They would then float the bonds, making their profits (reckoned to be a cool £40 million in the case of the Turkish issues) if the market paid a higher price than the percentage actually passed over to the issuers. But the countries involved were still left with a debt reflecting the face value of the bonds they had issued, not the sum they had actually received. Even the Costa Ricans, reckoned a good credit risk, owed £2.4 million after a bond issue from which they received a mere £700,000, or less than a third of the total.

The Costa Ricans were part of what might be called the 'sphere of influence' of the most remarkable of all the imperialist buccaneers, C. Minor Keith. Keith was a crucial figure in the history of indirect imperialism. His beginnings were heroic. In emulating the efforts of his uncle Henry, he pressed ahead with building railways in Central America even after his three brothers had all died of tropical diseases. But he ran out of funds after completing only 100 km (60 miles) of the tracks of what he had hoped would be a complete railway system for the region linking the Atlantic and Pacific coasts. Forced to find another source of revenue, he planted an experimental estate of bananas, and after a first shipment quickly sold out on its arrival in New Orleans he expanded his plans to cover much of Honduras and Guatemala with banana plantations.

The growing success of his banana empire, which he named United Fruit, reduced his interest in a railway through the length and breadth of Central America. Indeed, and ironically given the origins of his interest in bananas as merely a means of financing the railway, United Fruit was rightly attacked for building only railways which connected its plantations with the coast, neglecting routes which would serve the major towns and cities of the countries where he was operating. Even today the lines in Honduras and Guatemala do not connect the countries' main cities with each other or with the sea.

Early on United Fruit realized that control over the primary means of transport conferred almost absolute power. Over a period of nearly a century the invariably weak national governments tried in vain to tie it down with contractual commitments to meet the needs of the local people rather than the company.

Yet Keith was no simple imperial ogre. He married the daughter of the President of Costa Rica and formed one of the world's best collections of Central American antiquities, so could never be accused of being the sort of mindless capitalist trampling over local ways who figured in anti-imperialist propaganda.

Honduras and Guatemala were perfect examples of the much-despised 'banana republics' which depended for their national income on a single cash crop, produced and marketed by a single foreign concern. But they were not the original model for the idea of a single-crop economy depending on railways. The need to transport sugar cane from the plantations in the heart of Cuba to the coast meant that within a few years the island had 4000 km (2500 miles) of standard gauge as well as 4000 km (2500 miles) of narrow gauge sugar lines, at a time when Jamaica, for instance, had less than a tenth of the mileage.

So it was the railways which set off an argument with which we are increasingly familiar: between a country's need for subsistence crops to enable it to feed itself, against the fact that financiers are prepared only to invest in cash crops which give the return (especially in hard, which means foreign, currency) required to justify the capital expenditure involved.

For, too often, the railways left a miserable legacy. In the words of a local lady talking to a foreign visitor (in Maria Soltera's *A Lady's Ride Across Spanish Honduras*, published in 1884):

We have had many misfortunes of late years, Señora ... and many bad examples from those who assume to teach us progress in commercial transactions. Just look at that Honduras railway! It might have made the country! Ah, Señora, we have to thank the British people for ruining our trade and commerce for many years to come.

6 Regions and Industries

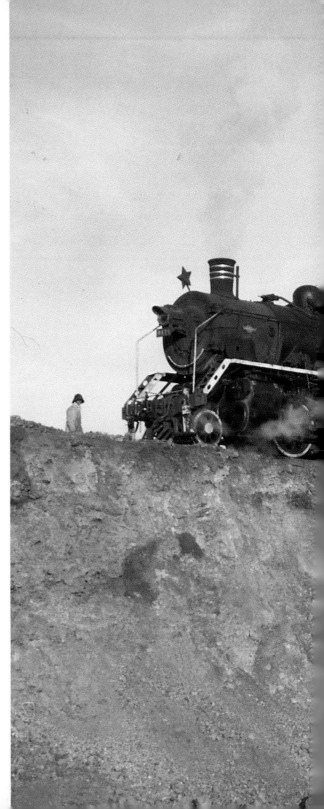

I n 'new' countries or regions the railways fulfilled every conceivable role: social, economic, political. The regions they created ranged from Florida to Manchuria. Only railways could open up Siberia, the Argentine pampas, the landlocked great plains of the United States, or the Canadian prairies to their north. In the second half of the nineteenth century these were transformed – thanks to the railways – into the greatest breadbaskets the world had ever seen. These provided the world's urban masses with an unprecedented supply of cheap grain – and, not coincidentally, ruined the British aristocracy by dramatically reducing the profit from their landholdings.

The Trans-Siberian, the longest of them all, was not the first imperialist Russian railway. That had been the railway to the Caspian Sea, built partly to counter British ambitions in central Asia, partly to demonstrate that Russia remained a Great Power, despite its defeat in the Crimean War. The Trans-Siberian itself, started in the late 1890s after decades of indecision, had several aims: to counter Japanese attempts to muscle in on the decay of the Chinese Empire further east; and, above all, to settle the vast Siberian plains and bring the far-flung existing communities together. Settling people in Siberia would, it was felt, also offset the land hunger and overcrowding in European Russia, which was naturally leading to unrest.

Steel and railways have always been intimately linked – as they are in Anshan Province in China today.

116

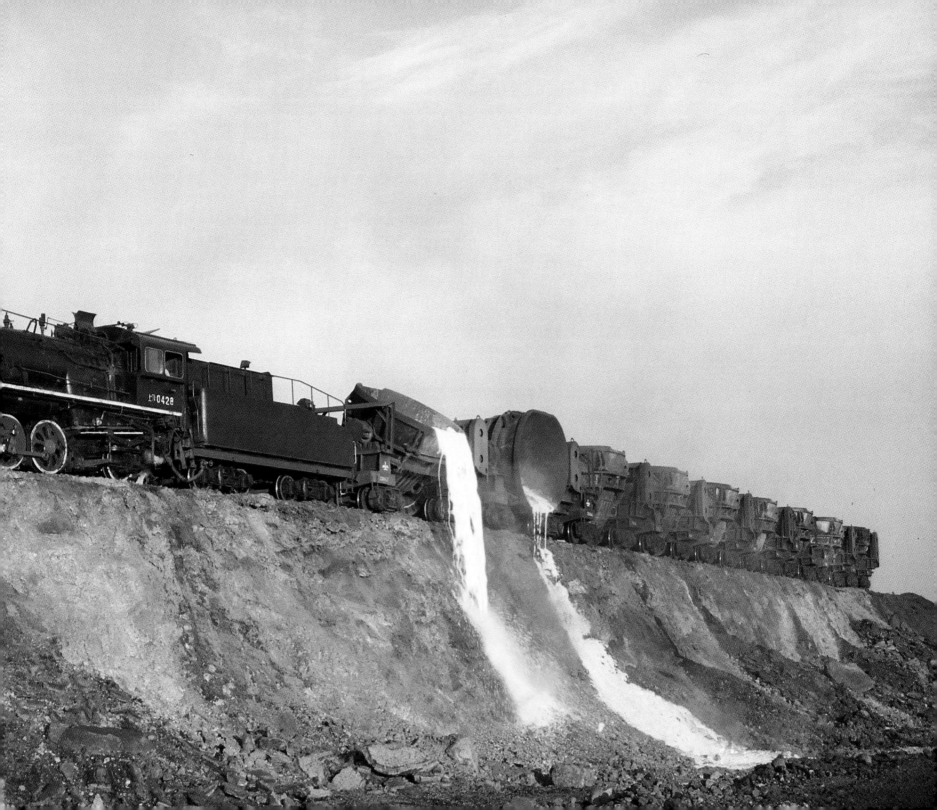

The Russians were also looking at the crumbling Chinese empire – hence the importance of the Chinese Eastern railway through Manchuria, which was only nominally Chinese. This line not only shortened the distance from Moscow to the Pacific, it also offered considerable commercial and military scope – although railways were perceived as so potent a weapon that merely building it triggered off the Russo-Japanese war, since the Japanese, not unnaturally, saw the arrival of the lines as a threat to their hopes of increasing their influence in the region.

In the late 1890s and early 1900s the Tsar's government made colossal efforts to encourage emigration to Siberia along the Trans-Siberian line, but without total success. Whole villages often travelled together, but many returned when they found that they could not cope with the climate or with having to defend themselves against the many violent criminals who had been exiled to Siberia together with the more-publicized but less numerous political criminals.

Yet most of the newcomers stayed and thrived. They not only grew wheat but fed grain to millions of cows to produce milk – and thus butter, a dairy product which could be transported over long distances. They were so successful that a limit had to be imposed on the export of butter, the famous Chelyabinsk Break, which imposed a tax on Siberian butter destined for Moscow passing west of the town.

Like Tsarist Russia, the United States was an 'invertebrate' economy before the coming of the railway. In particular, there were only the most exiguous links between the gigantic river systems of the Mississippi and Missouri and the states on the Atlantic seaboard, themselves strung along a thousand miles of coastline. Indeed, until the railways conquered the Appalachians, the cities' hinterlands were confined to the, often rather narrow, coastal belt. The only exception, the Erie Canal, proved the desperate need for proper routes, because it gave New York such a lead. Clearly every other major trading centre was going to seize on the railway as a means to emulate the example set by the Big Apple.

So every major city, notably rival seaports on the Atlantic coast like Boston, New York and Baltimore, fought to ensure that they had the best (and earliest) railway communications with their hinterland. Later, when the tracks reached beyond the

Mississippi, numerous were the complaints – usually justified – that promoters of new lines would bypass existing settlements unless they were paid a handsome sum of money in advance. The threat was no joke: the Mormon capital, Salt Lake City, was left stranded nearly a hundred miles from the first transcontinental route.

For the railways saved the United States from the tyranny imposed by the capricious flow of its river system. The train's precursors and theoretically its greatest rivals, steamships on canals, rivers and lakes, suffered from one crucial disadvantage: they depended on the vagaries of nature, on the whimsical directions taken by navigable water, and by the fact that so much of it iced up in winter, or dried up in summer. For even apparently untroubled rivers like the upper Mississippi (or the Rhône), were, in reality, if not impassable, exceptionally tricky to navigate because of shoals, shallows, or obstructions. Even in temperate climates, even in supposedly developed countries, railways had enormous seasonal advantages. In Mediterranean countries, they were unaffected by the heavy autumn rains which turned roads in Spain or Italy into impassable seas of mud.

As in Siberia, so in the Americas, the new regions needed settlers, and these were both transported and encouraged by the railways. The railway companies brought Italians to work on the pampas, and Germans and above all hardy Scandinavians, used to long, cold winters, to people the northern prairies. They encouraged emigration by employing agents along the whole route from Europe, through the emigrants' port of entry (usually Boston or New York), to their eventual destination.

The competition between the American railways for suitable settlers was ferocious. Perhaps the most cherished group was the Mennonites, Germans who had been settled in the Crimea for over a hundred years and were especially favoured because they were famously efficient farmers. In the end the Santa Fe captured them, but at such cost that, in modern terms, they were a 'loss-leader' for the railway. North of the border the Canadian Pacific was luckier, since it had a monopoly, and settled over fifty thousand families in hundreds of small settlements throughout the prairies. But usually the railways had to be pioneers themselves. Only occasionally was there existing traffic for them to build on, as could the Santa Fe when it followed the old-established cattle trails which linked the great plains with Omaha and, above all, with Chicago.

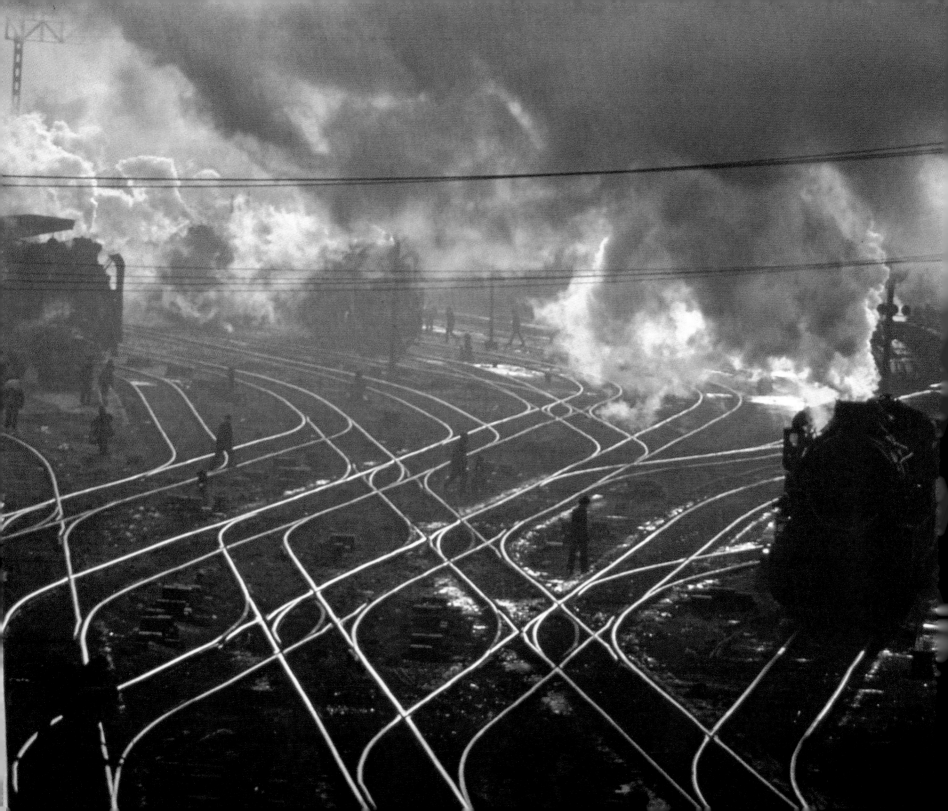

The CPR and the American railways needed the settlers with special urgency, for the companies' financing depended on their ability to sell the strips of land along the tracks which had been granted to them as part of their charters. But the promoters were walking a tightrope. They had to persuade potential investors that the land grants were a potential goldmine, while at the same time assuring legislators, the press and the public that the very same tracts were virtually worthless.

Both ideas could be true. Sometimes – most notably with the Central Pacific from Northern California into the High Sierras and the Rockies – the grants were of barren, mountainous strips of land, worthless even after the tracks had been built. In many other instances the grants seemed excessively generous, especially to later generations. The 'grant element' was so important that the Illinois Central, the first line to exploit its concessions on a large scale as early as the 1850s, was regarded by the stock market as a 'land company with a railway attached.' But the most obvious instance was the Union Pacific, the pioneering transcontinental route, which traversed the empty, fertile great plains in its drive to meet the Central Pacific.

In fact the shareholders of the major companies did not benefit greatly from the grants of land, which generally had to be sold off while the line was being built to provide the necessary finance. The major beneficiaries were the railways' managers and directors who bought up the patchwork strips of land and merged them into larger and more profitable units. The same pattern had prevailed earlier in Britain where the railways were not allowed to buy land. But the country solicitors who drew up the railways' plans were able to buy cheaply in advance land they knew would jump in value once it was served by the railway.

In the United States the promoters of short lines often did better, for they were able to exploit particularly profitable connections, through a fertile valley or to an existing town. Similarly today in the United States their successors are finding that they can make better profits from specialized traffic than can the larger networks.

The descendants of the early settlers still remember their roots, and the why and how of their journeys to their present homes. Ruth Kugler's family came from Germany, lured by the railways' advertisements in local papers and handbills which 'made all kinds of

Left *The Chinese relied on steam power – used intensively – long after the rest of the world had abandoned it.*

Overleaf *The modern paradox: motor manufacturers rely on trains to transport their products to their customers – in this case in Germany.*

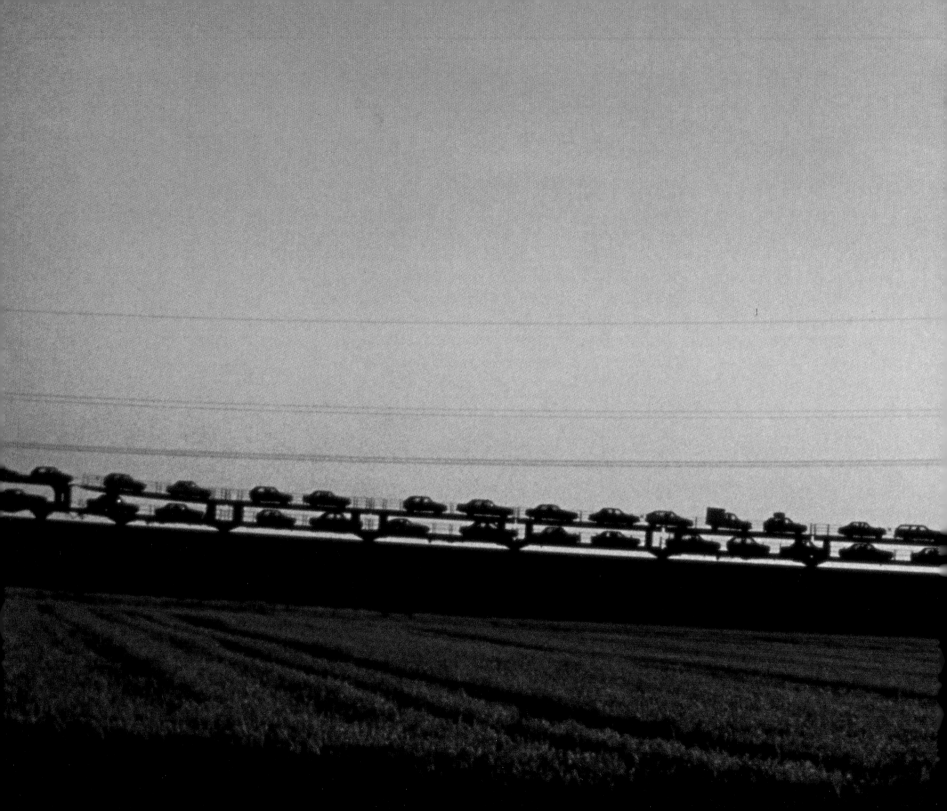

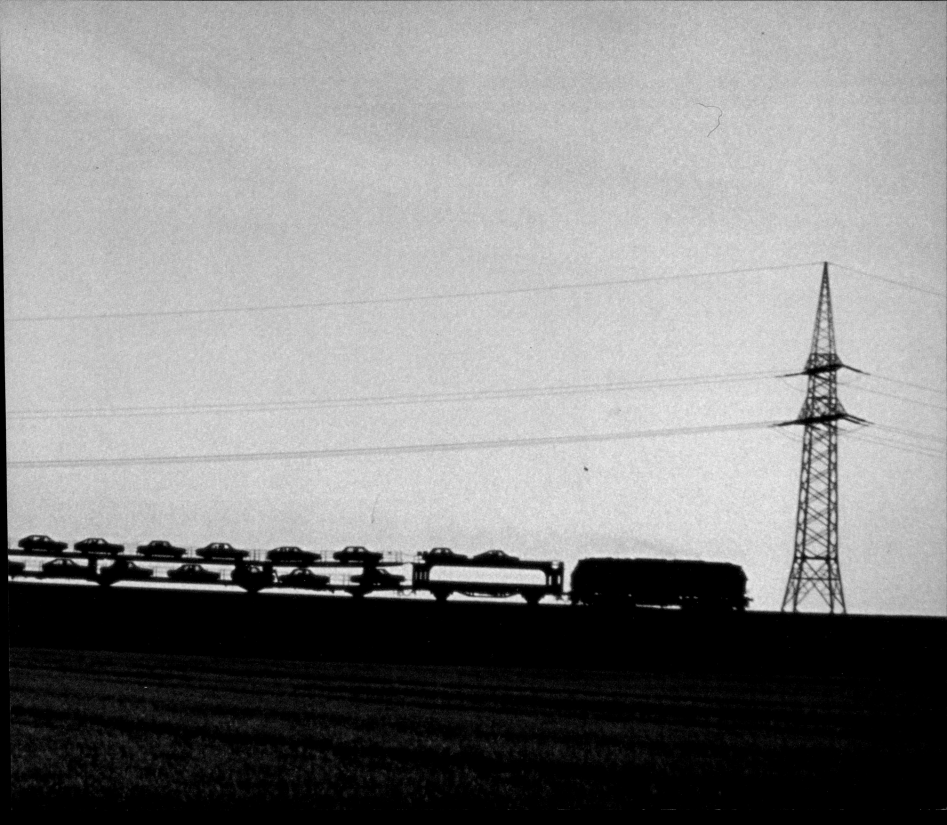

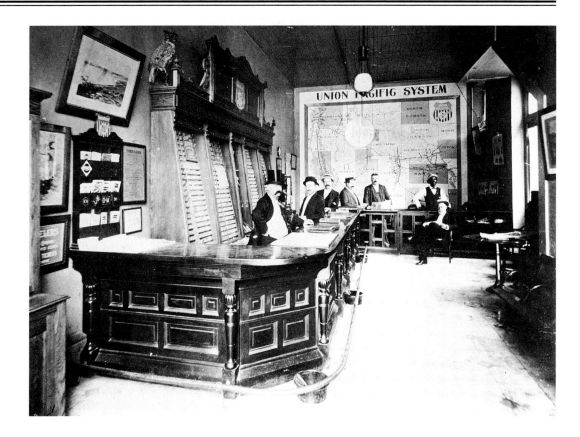

The opulence of the trappings in a booking hall on the Union Pacific emphasizes the dignity of everything connected with the railways.

Opposite top In Nebraska – as everywhere west of the Mississippi – trains were the universal providers, carrying everything from passengers to farming machinery.

Opposite below Tourist class on the Canadian Pacific: some comfort, more overcrowding.

promises that life in the new land would really be great … Germany was having political problems at the time and the land was becoming crowded.'

As late as 1922, Janet Kuska's father, the last colonization agent employed by the Burlington Railroad, 'went back east and actually recruited people to come back to the Midwest and to settle along the railway lines.' Jim Ehrenberger, who used to work for the Union Pacific, recalls how the immigrants arrived. 'They came in what were called immigrant cars. In fact they had a nickname for them, they called them "Zulu cars" … One end of it had the livestock and maybe some farm machinery. The other end had the household goods and the people would ride right in that car.' Once they reached their destination, says Janet Kuska:

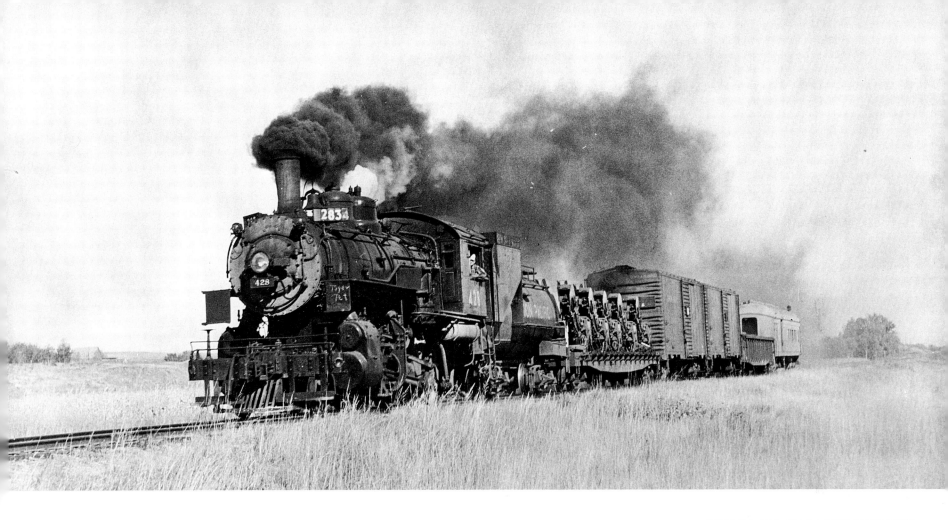

... they would either sell them at a very cheap rate, or in some instances they homesteaded the land ... if they prospered the railway prospered because they would ship their things on the railway ... the desirable people they were looking for were those that they knew would be successful. And they'd know they'd be successful by personal interviews ... The weather in the Midwest is a little rough and sometimes the situation is a little isolating ... so they had to look for those who really had the stick-to-itiveness and who were going to work the land and going to do a good job.

It was a hard life. Ruth Kugler remembers how the family had only a 'sodhouse', made of the local mud. 'My grandmother had several barrels outside of the sodhouse door. These she filled with snow so that she would have water for cooking and washing.'

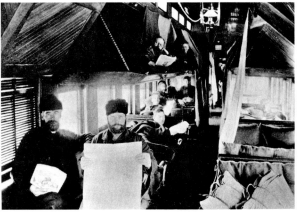

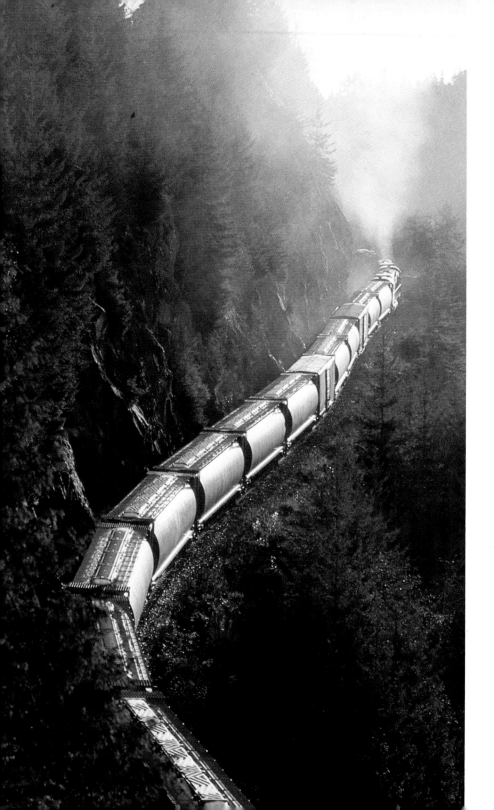

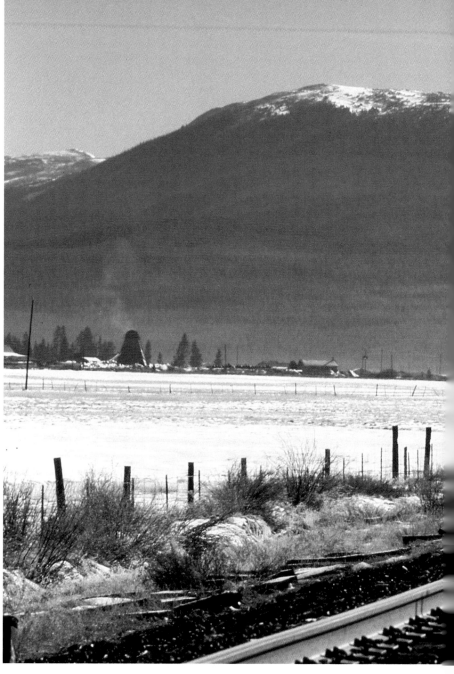

Left *Howe Sound in British Columbia – the routes through the Canadian Rockies are spectacular, but less well-publicized – than those in the United States*

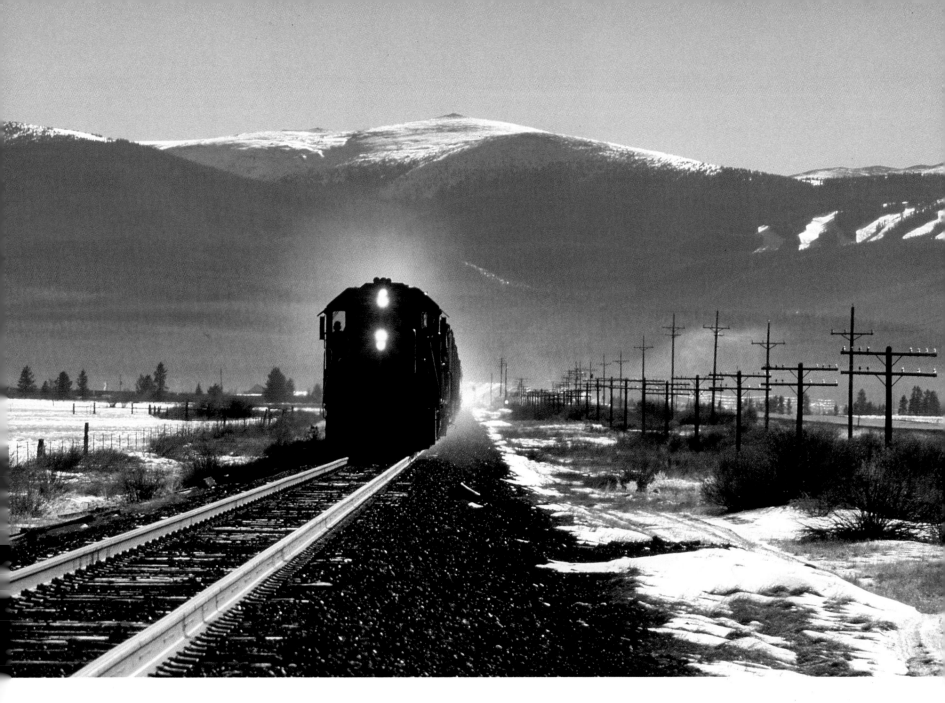

Above *The Rockies in Colorado make an incomparable backdrop for the railroad passenger.*

One settler with the requisite qualities was Bill Robb. His great-grandson Joe Jeffrey, who still farms part of his forebear's land, recounts how Robb had bought land from the Union Pacific. At first he didn't have an easy time. He was of Scottish-Irish extraction but surrounded by Scandinavians: 'The Swedes didn't like him ... because he was a brazen type. A big man, 6 ft 4 in, and he got his way most of the time.'

He was clearly not an easy man. He quarrelled with the Union Pacific, preferring to drive his cattle a few extra miles to the Burlington system: '... and when he died in Omaha the specific instructions were that his body was not to be delivered back to the gravesite out at the ranch by the Union Pacific, it must be brought back by the Burlington.' Jeffrey remembers shipping the cattle live on Sunday in time for the Monday markets in Chicago and Kansas City 'Sundays was a great event round here. We would all gather down to the stockyards and load train after train. And it seemed to me as a youngster that we just never got through loading cattle.'

Once the settlers had arrived the railways' job changed, with the colonization agent turning into an agricultural agent and educator, as Janet Kuska remembers:

> On the Burlington they would have trains on swine production to show how to produce a better hog, and they would have lime trains to show how to use that in farming. They also had what they called a smut train [which people mistook for a train carrying loads of pornography] but it was really something to do with wheat and the disease that wheat would get.

They even had a funeral procession, complete with a casket, mourners and a clergyman to read a service, all mourning the death of one Timothy Hay. 'The idea was that they wanted people to plant alfalfa instead of timothy ... and they wanted people to cultivate timothy into the ground so that it would act as a fertilizer.'

North of the border William Van Horne of the Canadian Pacific followed much the same policy. He built enormous grain elevators to protect the quality (and thus the reputation) of the hard wheat grown along the CPR's tracks, particularly in Manitoba, and encouraged the settlers to grow more suitable strains of wheat – one of which, Red Fife, he carried free. The CPR's more northerly competitor, the Canadian National, encouraged the development of Marquis, a new strain of wheat which would grow a hundred miles further north than existing varieties. Indeed suitable strains of wheat were crucial – the great appeal of the Mennonites was not only that they were disciplined and hard-working but that they brought with them a valuable strain of wheat called Turkey.

But regional development was not confined to the prairies. Only the northern half of Florida had been settled until the construction of the railway down the east coast. This was the work of Henry Flagler, a key partner of John D. Rockefeller in the creation of Standard Oil. He not only created the state in its modern form, but also the two industries on which it has depended ever since: tourism and citrus-growing. He and the railway remained deeply involved in the state's economy – after a devastating frost during the winter of 1884–85 he secretly spent a great deal of money helping the orange-growers get back into full production. He even instituted a regular system of weather forecasts and frost warnings. At times of danger the locomotive engineers would sound six long blasts on their whistles as they passed the threatened orchards.

But a region transformed by the arrival of the railway did not have to be exotic or previously uninhabited. In England, Cornwall had long been almost a separate kingdom, stranded far to the west of the rest of the country before Brunel's last great triumph, the Saltash Bridge over the Tamar river, brought the railway to the Duchy. It revolutionized Cornwall's economy, carrying hundreds of thousands of tourists in the summer and enabling it (and the Scilly Isles to the west) to benefit from their early spring. London could be supplied with spring flowers and early vegetables brought overnight by rail to Covent Garden. In 1896 alone an unbelievable 514 tonnes of flowers left Penzance Station for the rest of the country. These new industries provided some compensation for the decline of tin and copper mining in the last third of the nineteenth century.

Only railways could provide a proper network binding a country together and thus endowing it with a unified economic system. This was important in France where the waterways flowed to the Atlantic, the Channel or the Mediterranean, resulting in a triple division. In particular, it took the creation of a through line between Paris and the

Mediterranean to end the isolation of Provence – and also to ensure that local merchants could not hold the population to ransom when there was any shortage of food.

In developed countries the railways often merely intensified existing traffic flows. Economically, socially, politically, they could never run against a country's grain. In Wales, for instance, the division between north and south was merely reinforced by the railways, which for obvious economic reasons tended to follow the existing traffic, along the south coast and from the coal-mining valleys to the ports on the Bristol Channel and along the north coast from Chester to Holyhead. Rail travel between north and south remains inconvenient even today. (Only the need to appease Welsh national feeling keeps the lines open.)

Before the railways every region tended to be self-sufficient, but their arrival encouraged economies of scale and thus industrial specialization. The result was a great sorting out with towns, villages or entire regions acquiring fame as homes of particular products, spelling the ruin of local industries elsewhere which had been sheltered by the cost of transport from distant, if more efficient rivals. With this specialization came concentration, either on existing centres, or on towns which acquired a new importance as a result of the blossoming of a rail-borne speciality, and this in turn led to the reduced importance of smaller towns. Growth was concentrated on the larger towns, those most likely to be served earliest and best by railways.

In Britain products as different (but, crucially, as heavy) as bricks and beer became nationally distributed. The vaults under St Pancras station were designed to enable them to store the barrels of beer brewed at Burton over a hundred miles away. A rhapsodic account of the life of a great London terminus published in *Railway News* in 1864 describes the arrival of trains bearing:

> Manchester packs and bales, Liverpool cotton, American provisions, Worcester gloves, Kidderminster carpets, Birmingham and Staffordshire hardware, crates of pottery from North Staffordshire and cloth from Huddersfield, Leeds, Bradford and other Yorkshire towns.

In the United States the railway buff Lucius Beebe, writing in *Mixed Train Daily* in 1947, sang of short lines which depended on a single product:

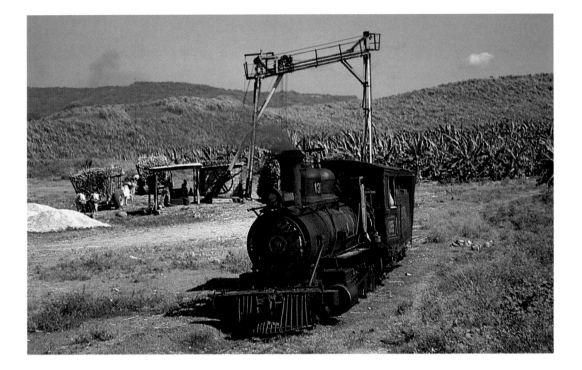

The Cubans are still using American-made engines to carry sugar cane to the coast on tracks laid before those in Spain, then Cuba's imperial master.

The dominant traffic of the Durham and Southern is Carolina tobacco, of the Clarendon and Pittsford the quarried marble of Vermont, and of the Bath and Hammondsport the wine grapes of upper New York. The Unadilla Valley lives almost alone by the dairy products of its region, and the Atlantic and East Carolina is known as 'The Mullet Line' by reason of the quantities of that fish it carries.

But the specialization bred by the railways was not only industrial. In France the vineyards in the south prospered and once they were able to deliver their strong *gros rouge* to Paris and the North they wiped out the vineyards which had existed since medieval times in Paris itself and round Orleans, where the growers turned to another speciality, vinegar. A number of land-locked wine districts, Saint-Emilion in France, Chianti in Tuscany, and the Rioja region of Northern Spain, found their proper place in the sun, or rather on the drinker's palate, thanks to the access to markets at home and abroad provided by the railways. And in Argentina, Italian immigrants in the land-locked province of Mendoza were able to produce vast quantities of wine to slake the thirst of the inhabitants of Buenos Aires hundreds of miles away. But then every country or region seemed to find an appropriate speciality. Butter from Holland (and from Normandy and the Charentes in western France) and bacon from Denmark became internationally-traded commodities.

So railways bred districts or whole regions entirely devoted to one type of produce, secure in the knowledge that the rest of their requirements could be paid for by their cash crop. Monoculture of grain was practised on the great plains in the United States, Canada and Russia from the start. But even existing agricultural areas were transformed, and not only by the new-found freedom from the previous need for a region to be self-sufficient.

In Spain a third of all the arable land in the country, originally needed to provide fodder for horses and draught oxen, was liberated by the arrival of the railways and could be used for growing grain. And in Spain, as elsewhere in the world (most obviously in the cattle country in the western prairies) animals no longer had to be driven to the slaughter-houses, losing weight and devouring every blade of grass in their path. They could be transported by train, ensuring that they arrived fit, fat (and, presumably, contented) at the abattoirs, leaving the pasture land untouched.

*I*n Britain most towns were quickly connected with main railway lines, and the same applied throughout continental Europe, if only because the promoters could not hope for a return on their investment unless they connected existing traffic centres. The economics of the line from Liverpool to Manchester, for example, depended on the line's capacity to compete with the (allegedly excessive) charges being demanded by the existing canal company. Like other early lines, the L&M was designed to tap existing freight traffic. So the promoters were often surprised by the extent of the previously unfulfilled demand for travel by individuals, either on business or for pleasure. Four hundred thousand people travelled on the L&M the year after it was opened, and within five years of its opening the London to Birmingham Railway was carrying a million passengers a year. Indeed all these and many other railway projects prefigured the situation familiar to more recent traffic forecasters, the failure to predict the popularity of such facilities as London's airports or the M 25 motorway.

The world's first proper railway system, between Stockton and Darlington, bred the first railway town, Middlesbrough, promoted by the same financiers who had provided the capital for the railway itself. They created a town and a port on a site which, before the railway was built, contained only a single farmhouse and its outbuildings. Yet within a couple of decades the town had twenty thousand inhabitants and was one of the busiest ports in the North of England. And by the mid-1840s the great Isambard Kingdom Brunel had established Swindon, the first town specifically created to cater for the railways' needs – as the place where they changed engines half-way between London and Bristol. But Swindon, and indeed the other 'railway towns' in Britain or abroad, were artificial constructs which never became major metropoli. Nor did the railways necessarily revolutionize existing towns which became major railway junctions. Bologna, for instance, was largely unaffected by its key position in the Italian railway system, and Olten, which fulfilled a similar role in central Switzerland, is still a relatively small town.

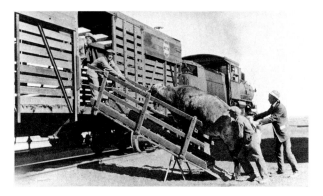

Plattner, Colorado: the reluctant animal seems to be aware that he is heading for the slaughter-houses of Chicago a thousand miles away.

In the United States the very pattern of settlement was determined by the fact that contemporary locomotives 'would only operate about a hundred miles at a time', in the words of Jim Ehrenberger, a former Union Pacific worker,

> ... and it usually took a full day to get across that hundred miles, especially with a freight train. And as a result they would set up a little terminal every hundred miles, and this terminal consisted not only of a station but it would have a hotel and an eating house and a round house and usually shops to repair the locomotive. And of course that's what also brought in manpower and caused some of the creation of some of these towns because it was the railway workers too that created the towns.

Towns were even moved to capture the advantages of being on the tracks. According to Joe Jeffrey the almighty Union Pacific told the inhabitants of Plum Creek that 'they wouldn't make a stop unless you move your town to one of our sections. And so in about 1882–3 the little town of Plum Creek was moved just to the west, about half a mile, so it would be on a railway.'

The number of new settlements was astonishing. The Santa Fe alone created so many that two hundred were named after employees of the railway company, and the Canadian Pacific gave birth to no fewer than eight hundred new towns and villages in its march

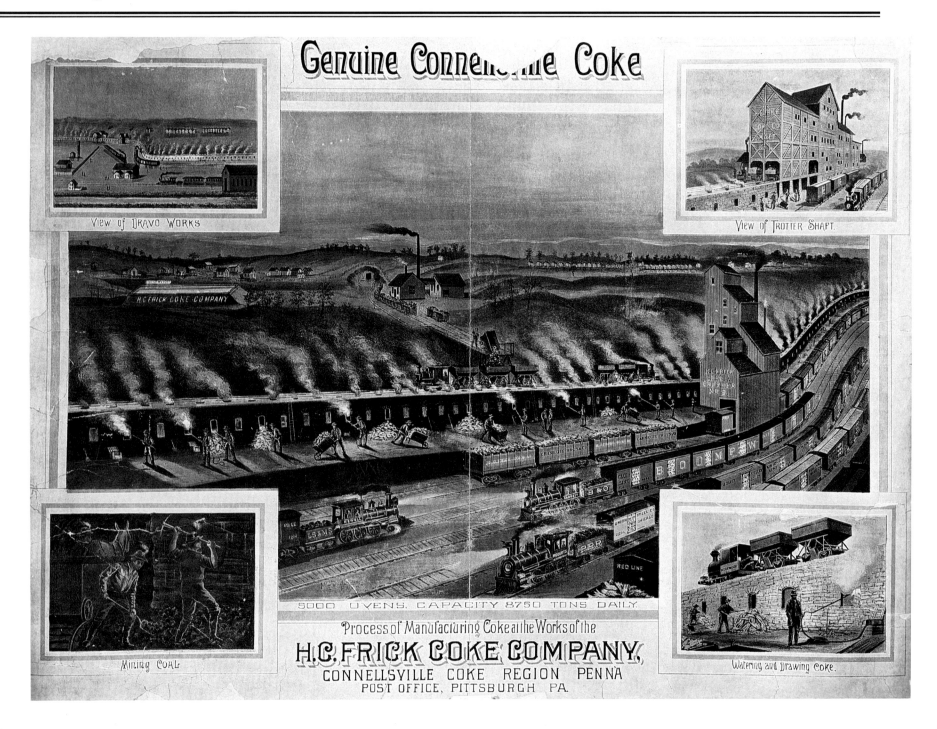

Genuine Connellsville Coke

View of DRAVO WORKS

View of TROTTER SHAFT.

Mining Coal.

Watering and Drawing Coke.

5000 OVENS, CAPACITY 8750 TONS DAILY.

Process of Manufacturing Coke at the Works of the

H. C. FRICK COKE COMPANY,

CONNELLSVILLE COKE REGION PENN'A

POST OFFICE, PITTSBURGH PA.

across the prairies. Of course many of them were purely temporary, the 'hells on wheels' which so fascinated American moralists because of the vice and violence which inevitably accompanied the onward march of the railway builders. But some of these dens of iniquity, like Cheyenne, soon settled down as permanent communities, no more or less law-abiding than cities with less disreputable origins.

But the most important urban development was not the railhead or the 'railway town' but the crucial point where a railway provided its hinterland, generally a major agricultural region, with access to navigable water. Indeed only two of the many major American cities founded in the nineteenth century (Denver and Indianapolis) were not on navigable waterways. The classic conjunction was Chicago, the dream city of the third quarter of the nineteenth century. Los Angeles, its equivalent a century later, is so well known for its worship of the motor car that its debt to the railways which brought the original immigrants to the 'City of the Angels' is now largely forgotten.

Chicago is on Lake Michigan and so it is connected with the other Great Lakes which provided an outlet to the Atlantic. Its prospects were transformed by the vital rail link to the Mississippi (at two points, Quincey, Illinois and Burlington, Iowa – hence the fame, and importance, of the Chicago, Burlington & Quincy railway) which brought together the two biggest water systems in the United States. In the words of Howard Rosen, the business historian, 'Chicago became the point between the agricultural west and the industrial and populous northeast.'

It was a romantic city which rejoiced in qualities which would have been a matter of shame in less self-confident communities. Les Orear, a veteran meatpacker and union organizer, admits that 'the city was just covered with soot. It was a sooty city.' But, 'the smoke and grime was just a part of big city life here in Chicago.' The poet Carl Sandburg was equally typical in romanticizing its very grimness: 'City of the big shoulders, hog butcher to the world.' This was entirely appropriate, for as Les Orear put it:

> The meatpacking industry, which was the pride and joy, the first great industry that took off here really, put Chicago on the map. As industry diversified, it created more and more products to be shipped out on the rails and the fact that the rails were there made it possible for Chicago to grow by leaps and bounds.

Opposite Henry Frick's Coking Plant: *a powerful symbol of the industrial might unleashed by the railways, and, suitably, the scene of one of the bitterest strikes in American history.*

For Chicago became, according to Rosen:

> ... a place where factories that produce for a national market would locate in – in agricultural implements, in steel, in textiles and manufactured goods, in a whole range of agricultural by-products, from the Armour and Swift of the meatpacking industries to the Sears Roebuck kind of catalogue.

Eventually 23 railways included the city's name in theirs. Howard Rosen explains that 'you had at least seven major transcontinental lines coming in. And you had two major beltways, one near north and one near south, that would serve the lighter, smaller industries that didn't have a direct service themselves.'

The stockyards were enormous. 'Think of it,' exclaims Les Orear, 'a mile square of stockyard pens, livestock move in in the morning, unloaded from the trains,' before being despatched to the slaughterhouse and thence, through a series of long chutes, to be dismembered in enormous complexes. 'In the Armour plant where I worked,' Orear remembers, 'there were approximately 72 buildings.'

Like the other processing plants it was on property owned by the Chicago Junction railway, most typical of the city's railways and designed primarily to service the meat-packing industry. The CJ had a symbiotic relationship with the meatpackers. 'The railways really ran the tempo of the shipping departments ... everything ran by the railway's requirement.' But the dependence was mutual. Faced by the threatened departure of the meatpackers, the CJ, as Howard Rosen explains, 'undertook a response which was perhaps typical of what railways did in that era. They planned a new development. They organized perhaps the first example of an industrial park, the Central Manufacturing District.' In the end there were several along the tracks, for the railways 'created factories, created streets, street lighting, the sewers, the sidewalks, every aspect including even medical care.'

George Pullman, who made his name synonymous with luxurious dining and sleeping cars, went even further, building a company town named after him on the outskirts of Chicago, housing fourteen thousand people and totally dependent on his company. But the accommodation reflected the corporate hierarchy, its size, location and quality depending on whether you could afford the rent. There was even a row of smaller units suitable for honeymoon couples. According to George Ryan,

> He gave the workers excellent housing but he dictated how they were to live, how they were to have their houses decorated. . . . The problems he caused were telling people how to live, where to sit and what to do with their free time. One instance is that if people sat on a porch in an undershirt, they were told not to sit around that way in public.

The dream was destroyed by the great slump of 1893.

> George Pullman went out and bid to make cars for other railways. And he underbid everybody and won the contract and then came back and told the workers that the good news was that his factory would remain open, the bad was that their wages would be cut.

But he wouldn't cut their rents, paid to a separate company which was pledged to maintain its six per cent dividend.

The result was a strike which spread to the railroads, where the workers, in solidarity with Pullman's employees, refused to operate his cars. In the end the strike was brutally suppressed with the help of federal troops, but it left a deep scar. Pullman's reputation was destroyed. He wasn't exactly broken, says Les Orear,

> . . . but he was reviled. He was afraid. The man was so afraid that when he died and was buried, he ordered that his grave be interlocked with rails welded together, bolted together to restrain grave robbers who might dig him up and desecrate him.

There was an Indian parallel to Pullman's town, if not his fate: Jamalpore in Bihar, deliberately developed well away from Calcutta and other sources of temptation and unrest, as a 'railway colony', a model imperial township. The facilities included neat and regular streets, centred around the aptly-named 'steam road' which was 'built on the most advanced principles of sanitary science'. It had its own armed police, its own brass band, Masonic lodge, two Christian churches and the other trappings of a Victorian town, like a proper library and a Mechanics' Institute. The races were carefully segregated, not only by the accommodation they were allotted, but according to ranks which were themselves determined by the worker's race.

But Pullman was only one suburb of a mighty city. Above all Chicago was big. In Howard Rosen's words:

> In Chicago what you see is scale . . . the national scale of industry that the railway brought is visible in the way Chicago developed and its emphasis on being first and being big. But it was not all stockyards and industrial estates. There's a legacy of bigness in Sears that you can see in the old Sears warehouse on the west side of Chicago.

Another 'big' Chicago innovation was the skyscraper, itself partly due to the engineering advances required by railways. As Howard Rosen points out,

> You couldn't have freight trains crossing rivers on cast iron . . . You needed steel . . . The consequent design [of the first bridge across the Mississippi], the use of structural steel, was taken by architects in Chicago, by Louis Sullivan in particular and the bridge was turned up on its axis and became the steel frame for the modern skyscraper. And so Chicago becomes the first place where the skyscraper is built in part because of the railway.

This tradition was reborn in the 1960s and culminated in the new Sears Tower in downtown Chicago, still the world's tallest office building.

Chicago was an unusual railway city, not only because its sheer size prevented it from being dominated by the railways, but because it was not reliant on coal traffic. For, in general, the railway and its trains were the by-products of the coal industry with which they retained a symbiotic relationship. This began with the steam pumps used in the mines; later the same type of engine was used for hauling loads to and from the coalface and then from the pit itself to the nearest navigable water. And the first railways were often developed because the owners of the canals were abusing their monopoly position – or, as in the case of the Stockton & Darlington, with a view to developing new collieries away from navigable water. Subsequently coal provided the base load for many

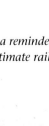

Chicago's famous 'El', a reminder that the railways obtruded into the very heart of the ultimate railway city.

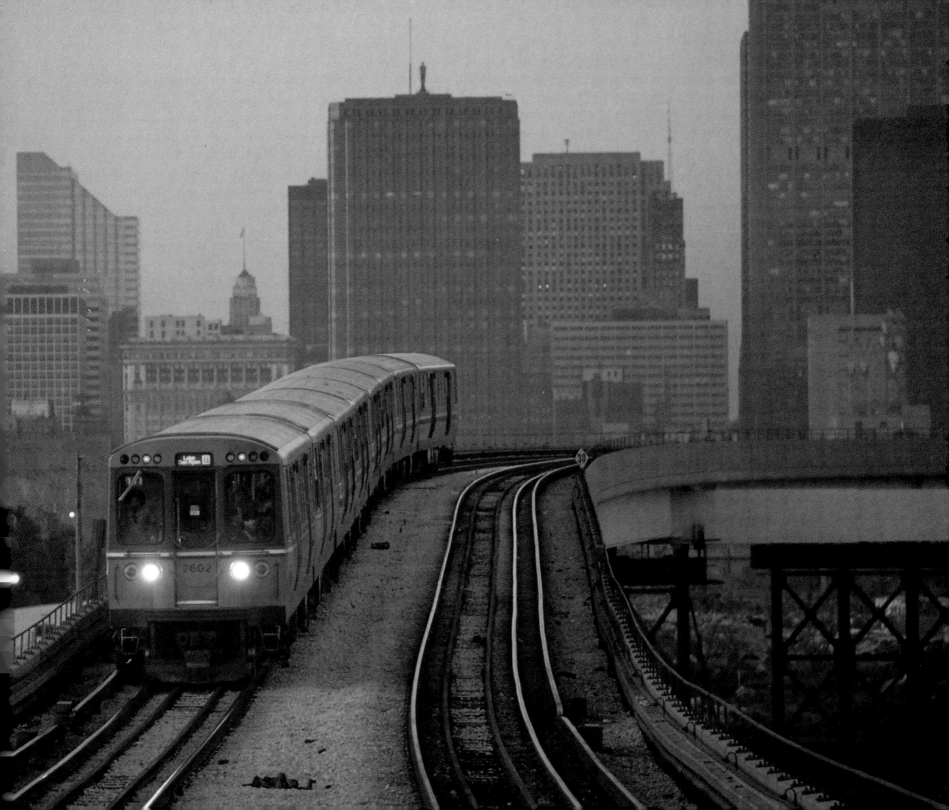

a railway – indeed when the American railways had been brought to their knees in the 1970s by generations of over-regulation they carried virtually nothing else.

But later came railways designed not for coal but for high-value merchandise requiring transport faster and more reliable than was possible with water transport – offering the same advantage that allowed air transport to edge its way into the freight market a century later.

Industrially, however, the railways were in a sense their own best – and most demanding – customer. They created their own infrastructure, a sort of mechanical magic carpet which absorbed vast quantities of capital, vast numbers of men, and unprecedented amounts of coal and iron, steel and other metals. The companies demanded new materials, stronger cast iron, steel instead of iron. Like the aerospace industry in the twentieth century, they kept the technologists on their toes by their insatiable demand for improvement in materials and techniques.

The effects of the industrial revolution sparked off by the railways increased over decades, even generations. Their contribution to the British economy nearly tripled in the quarter of a century after 1865 – by which time most of the country's network had already been in existence for a decade or more – and the same cumulative effects can be seen elsewhere in the world.

Steam had powered the first industrial revolution, in the form of the spinning-jennies of Lancashire. Steam power on wheels proved crucial to development elsewhere. Outside North America the most striking instance of an economy transformed by the railways is Germany, an astonishingly backward country until the middle of the nineteenth century. In the newly-uniting country railways were the prime instrument of industrialization. In the Ruhr they built on their original role, that of linking coal mines with navigable water, and in Germany as a whole railways accounted for a quarter of the total industrial investment. The need for rails (imported from England for some time) spurred on the development of the steel industry. Alfred Krupp's success was largely due to the development of springs, rails, and steel wheels for railway locomotives and wagons stronger than any made before – expertise which proved handy when making cannons. This was normal elsewhere. As Albro Martin notes (in *Railroads Triumphant*), in its early years:

Making rails was what the American steel industry was all about, or nearly so ... the railways not only made the modern iron and steel industry possible by solving its transportation problems; as a market for the product, they also made it necessary. Their evolutionary histories remain inextricably intertwined.

For railways, important in themselves, were also pioneers of what might be called industrial synergy. They greatly increased the effect of another major invention, the Wheatstone telegraph, as well as the effectiveness of steam-powered ships. So, not surprisingly, countries measured their industrial success by the progress they made in building and operating railways and their associated locomotives and equipment – much of which had originally had to be imported from Britain.

Development was helped by the fact that locomotives needed repair and maintenance, so that even countries which imported them developed their expertise by repairing them. Then practice made perfect. It took the Japanese nearly forty years to eliminate the need to import steam locomotives, but they started producing electric locomotives less than a decade after the Germans, the first into the business.

But then the railways themselves were so much the most important industry in any country that their technological influence could extend into all sorts of unexpected directions: the first practical diving suit, for example, was used during the struggle to excavate the Severn tunnel, and railway tunnellers remained its most important customers for a generation or more; and on a lighter note Beyer-Peacock, the locomotive manufacturers responsible for so many of the engines used in the Third World, introduced photographs into their catalogues as early as 1856, the first time they had been used for publicity purposes. The railways' tentacles were everywhere.

7 Steam and Society

From the outset railways were thought of as progressive, democratizing institutions. The feeling was natural, since they carried rich and poor alike. In the stirring words of a speaker at the Internal Improvements convention held in New York in 1836: 'The railroad is the poor man's road. It is the rich man's money expended for the benefit of himself and the poor man.'

The feeling was summed up in the words of Dr Thomas Arnold when he saw a train passing Rugby School. He was overjoyed 'to see it and think that feudality is gone for ever. It is so great a blessing to think that any one evil is really extinct.' Ironically his sentiments were echoed by the reactionary Emperor Francis II of Austria who opposed the development of railways within his empire because they would bring in democratizing influences, what he described as 'rebellion'. In the event his successors found that railways' subversive influence was less important than their usefulness in helping to bind together their dominions, and as we saw in Chapter 4, in controlling them through facilitating troop movements. Politically, in other words, they were neutral.

Socially they were more effective, though railways could not by themselves reform societies or break the habits of centuries. The effects were patchy and varied from country to country. One simple but obvious example is the provision of railway services on the Sabbath. In the United States the railroads were powerful enough to impose their Sabbath-breaking will on small towns. The railroad at Galesburg, wrote Ernest Almo Calkins, in *They Broke the Prairie* in 1937, 'was no longer a neighborhood enterprise, controlled by the little group of pious men who had founded Galesburg to be a Christian town after their own ideal.'

In Britain rail services helped to erode the rigours of the traditional Protestant British

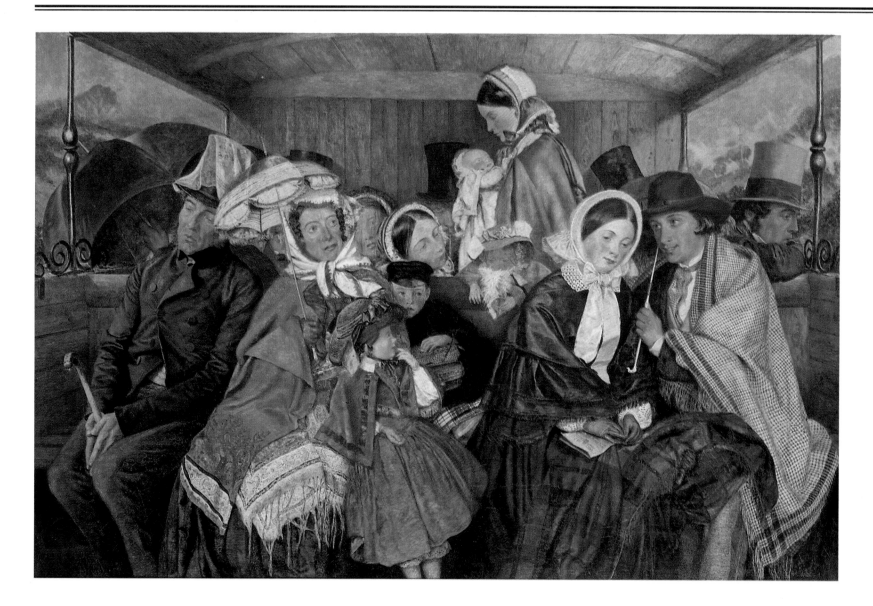

*The cramped reality of early excursion trains as
depicted by Charles Rossiter in his famous
'To Brighton and Back for 3s and 6d'.*

Sabbath – even though the Victorian Sunday coexisted with them. British railways have always had special timetables for Sundays, offering services which are invariably less fast and frequent than those of weekdays, whereas in continental Europe timetables are virtually the same throughout the week.

The Victorian era is generally thought of as a time of feminine enslavement, but contemporaries believed that the railways had greatly helped to free women. In 1844 an eminently respectable periodical, the *Quarterly Review*, noted with approval how the railways had brought about a change: 'the emancipation of the fair sex, and particularly of the middle and higher classes, from the prohibition from travelling in public carriages, which with the majority was a prohibition from travelling at all.' This new-found freedom was extended by the fact that many compartments on trains were mixed (although railways provided ladies-only compartments until well after 1945).

Typical of the way railways could encourage natural social trends but fail to shake older-rooted habits was in education. For a generation or more railways were thought of as the highest and most challenging form of construction. In Russia cadet engineer officers deemed it a great honour to work on the country's first main line, from Moscow to St Petersburg – although the young Fyodor Dostoyevsky was denied the honour because he somehow neglected to include any doors or windows in the fortress he designed as part of his studies.

In pre-railway days the military academy at West Point was the only one offering advanced technical studies in the United States. But in the 1840s and 1850s numerous schools were opened to satisfy the apparently insatiable demand for trained railroad engineers, and after the boom ended they broadened their curriculum to supply the country with well-trained engineers of every description. In France the railways' requirements merely reinforced the Napoleonic tradition, enshrined in elite institutions like the Ecole Polytechnique and the Ecoles des Ponts et Chaussées and Mines, that France's brightest should be trained to take charge of the most technologically advanced projects. Their skills were used to build railways, not only in France but in Spain, the Hapsburg Empire, and much of the rest of continental Europe as well, railways furnished by fellow-graduates with locomotives and equipment they had themselves designed.

In Britain, despite the sometimes exaggerated respect accorded to Brunel and the Stephensons, the country's education system for decades remained hermetically sealed to any suggestion that engineering was a subject entitled to the same respect as the Classics. But the British railway companies retained a greater sensitivity to their passengers' wishes, running more frequent, more regular (and usually faster) services than were available on the Continent, at least until the First World War. Indeed the race for the fastest trains at the time was generally between the British and the Americans. The first trains to travel at more than 100 mph ran on the Great Western Railway and the New York Central, a line which, in terms of average speeds, more than held its own with its expresses from New York to Atlantic City.

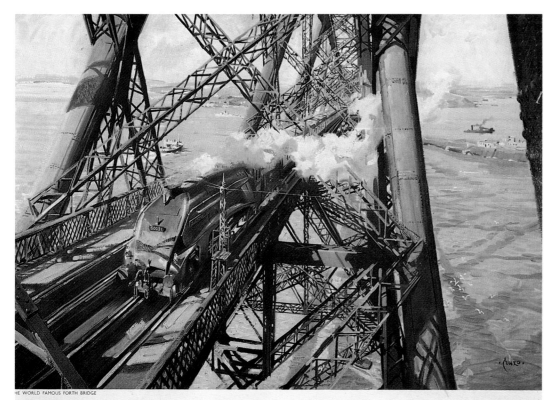

THE WORLD FAMOUS FORTH BRIDGE

SCOTLAND FOR YOUR HOLIDAYS

Nostalgia, British-style. Even after the railways were nationalized they used Terence Cuneo's romantic vision of the Flying Scotsman as publicity material.

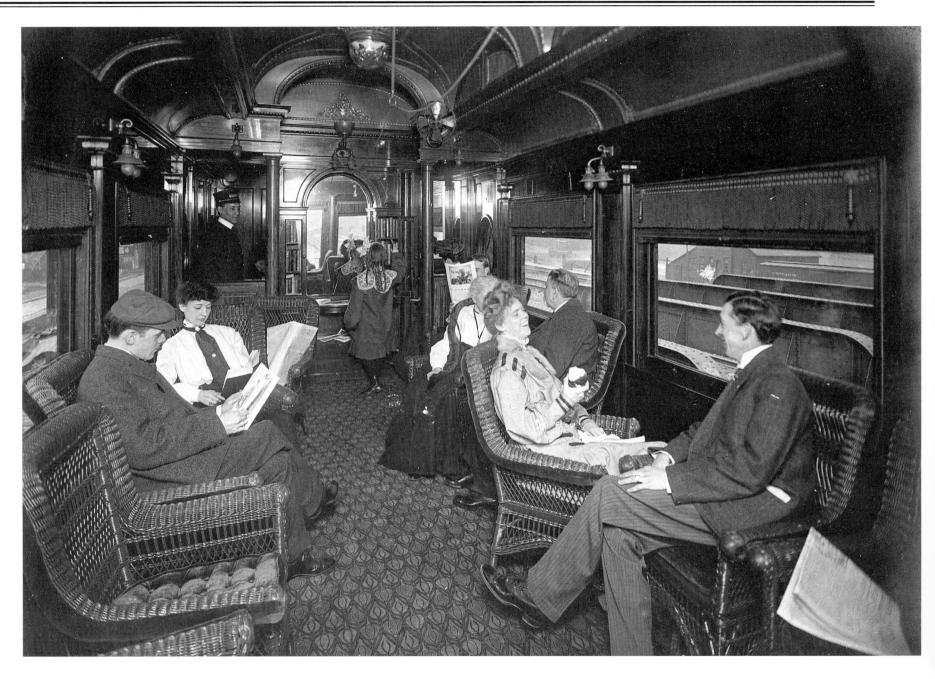

By contrast the French used to provide only a single daytime train from Paris transporting passengers to any important city in the provinces. There were more trains at
night but these were incredibly slow, and the service between provincial cities was
appalling – as late as 1951 it took a full day and night to travel by train from Brittany to
Lyon or the Mediterranean.

*C*lass structures remained – although, superficially, they *appeared* to change. In his
novel *Mr Facey Romford's Hounds*, R. S. Surtees, a railway enthusiast, wrote: 'all
people are put so much upon a par by the levelling influence of the rail, that a versatile
man may pass for almost anybody he likes – a duke, a count, a viscount.' He appeared
to have a point: the aristocracy soon abandoned their initial practice of mounting their
carriages on flat cars attached to the trains and started to travel in the same compartments
as their inferiors – albeit only those who could afford first-class fares. But, in their usual
contradictory fashion, the railways eliminated another type of personal contact: that
inevitable when travelling by road.

For mere contact did not necessarily weaken class structures. It made no difference
that upper-class Hindus travelled in the same trains, indeed in the same class of accommodation, as the lower orders. The gulfs between India's many castes remained totally
unaffected. Moreover from the very beginning the railways divided the accommodation
they provided into distinct classes. The lower orders travelled on hard benches in the
smoke and smut-filled carriages just behind the engine – indeed until the 1840s third-
class accommodation consisted only of open boxcars attached to freight trains. Gladstone's 1844 Act required them to be covered but they still looked more like boxcars
than true passenger carriages. From the start their betters travelled in more expensive –
and upholstered – comfort behind. Railways were an example of the way mechanical
improvements widened the opportunities for money to purchase luxury or speed, or
both, while not greatly affecting underlying social realities.

For, as so often, the railways reflected, rather than altered, class structures. Ironically,
railways in Britain, supposedly the most class-conscious of societies, never had more
than three classes. By contrast most Continental countries had four – and in the 1870s

Opposite *The Golden Age of American
rail travel, enough to arouse nostalgia
in the stoniest of hearts.*

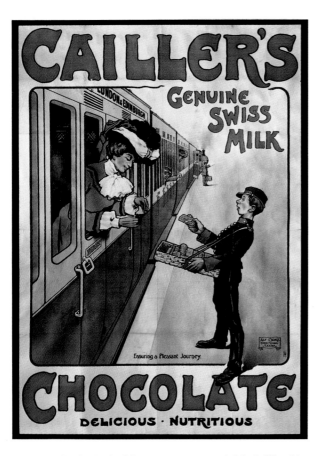

In the United States entrepreneurial lads like this, on a 1901 poster by Ney, were called 'news butchers' though their offerings were not confined to newspapers.

Opposite Profitable nostalgia: the Orient Express, still running after over a century.

the great Midland railway abolished the second class, a democratic step followed, albeit only slowly and reluctantly, by the other major companies.

American railways continued the tradition set on their steamboats, of having open carriages with an aisle (which some people referred to as 'the elongated spittoon') down the middle. This arrangement was widely perceived as an expression of the open, democratic spirit prevailing in God's own Republic, in contrast to the stuffiness and restrictiveness of older societies characterized by the closed compartments and rigid class system prevailing in Europe. But, what with coaches and parlour cars, the Americans soon developed a hierarchy of accommodation of their own (not forgetting the segregation automatically imposed on black people for over a hundred years). Other countries were more truly democratic – although Norway may be the only country which has never had any form of class distinction at any time in the history of its railways.

Other class distinctions soon emerged in terms of speed. Characteristically the Parliamentary trains – imposed on the railway companies by a Parliament anxious to enable the working classes to travel by train at reduced fares – soon became synonymous, not just with lack of comfort, but lack of speed as well. At the other extreme came the 'Limiteds', the glamorous trains which took precedence over all other traffic. Naturally these trains involved higher fares. But, as with aeroplanes, the real status attached to having your own transport. In Britain 'specials' could be chartered, and doing so symbolized urgency as well as power and wealth – Sherlock Holmes was for ever commanding Dr Watson to hire one. But they were thought a bit flash – Winston Churchill was considered frightfully extravagant when he hired one for election purposes in 1910.

In the United States power consisted not only in the ownership of 'specials' but also in their owners' ability to 'ride special', to override the existing pecking order in a railroad's operational scheme of things. There is a marvellous description of such an exercise in Kipling's *Captains Courageous* when the railroad tycoon, Cheyne, rushes across the continent to be reunited with the son he had supposed lost at sea.

Private cars were a suitable symbol of the Gilded Age in the United States, available not only for the native rich but also for travelling stars – Lillie Langtry, the actress and mistress of Edward VII, had her car painted Jersey Blue to match her eyes and her

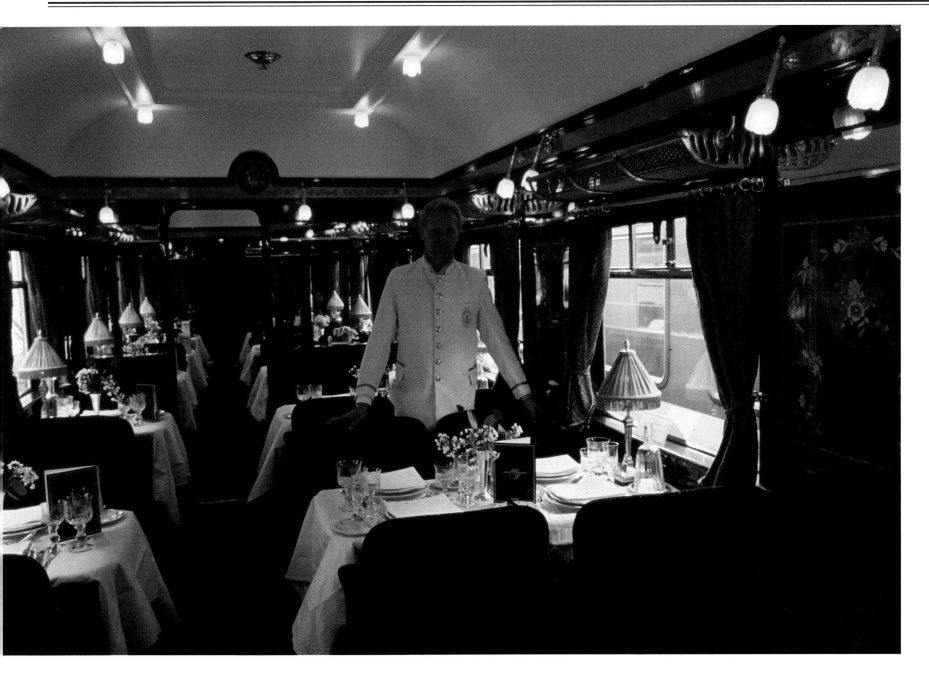

nickname, the Jersey Lily. But perhaps the most extraordinary such vehicle was one owned by the banker, Auguste Belmont: he had a special car of his own on the New York subway which he had helped finance.

Some complete train services were also seen as glamorous and exciting: this feeling was encouraged by a generous dollop of publicity from the operators, who showed clearly that hype is not a modern invention. In the United States the named trains included such wonders as the Cannonball, which Casey Jones was driving from Chicago to New Orleans the fatal night when he died trying to catch up on an hour's delay, and the Twentieth Century Limited, famous for its all-night poker games and the stars photographed alighting from it in Los Angeles.

Britain had the Flying Scotsman and the Cornish Riviera, the French had the Blue Train down to the Real Riviera. In Switzerland the Glacier Express ('the world's slowest express train') took the rich and famous up into Alpine ski resorts like St Moritz and Gstaad which had been tiny villages before the arrival of the railway. The track was so steep that the train's luxurious restaurant car was provided with wine glasses with slanted bases to ensure that they remained level even on the steepest incline.

The cult of the glamorous train was summed up in the Orient Express which first connected Paris with the mysterious Orient in 1883 – although for some years the last leg to Constantinople was traversed by sea. The promoter was a canny Belgian called Georges Nagelmackers, a pioneer in providing international sleeping car services (using carriages with German-designed bogies which provided a far smoother ride than wheels mounted on axles). He naturally ensured that the maiden voyage of the train was well publicized, since among the travellers were a well-known Parisian man of letters, Edmond About, who wrote a book about his experience, and Henri von Blowitz, the self-styled 'King of Journalists' who took the opportunity to interview the King of Romania, and scooped the world with the first-ever interview with the Turkish Sultan, Abdul Hamid.

In the following fifty years the train became a byword for international crime, intrigue and sex, the scene of innumerable thrillers (most obviously Graham Greene's *Stamboul Train* and Agatha Christie's *Murder on the Orient Express*). There were even real-life romances, as when the notorious arms dealer Sir Basil Zaharoff met the only love of his

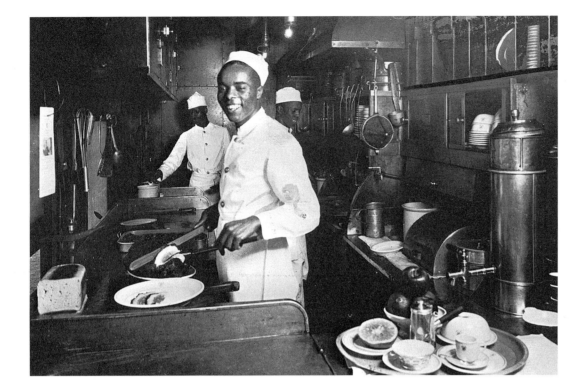

Preparing a hearty breakfast for travellers on the legendary Broadway Limited, which took a mere 20 hours to cover the 943 miles (1517 kms) from New York to Chicago.

evil life on the train (appropriately she was a Spanish duchess suffering at the hands of a cruel husband). After 1945 the original declined into an uncomfortable train meandering through the Balkans with a load of impoverished students, but the name was still so powerful that it was revived to attract a clientele for a train made up of the old rolling stock and used as a nostalgic journey into a (not entirely imaginary) past.

Luxury extended to the food served on the journey or at the stations – though not in Britain where the railway sandwich acquired an evil reputation within a few years, largely because the railways leased their refreshment rooms to entrepreneurs anxious to maximize their profits from a captive clientele. In France, by contrast, the buffets at such stations as the Gare de Lyon in Paris were associated with some of the country's finest food. Today, curiously, the situations have been reversed. France, with one of the finest train systems in the Western world, has very poor railway food, while BR's sandwiches are far better – indeed they are the same as those sold by Marks and Spencer, a fact many people find difficult to believe.

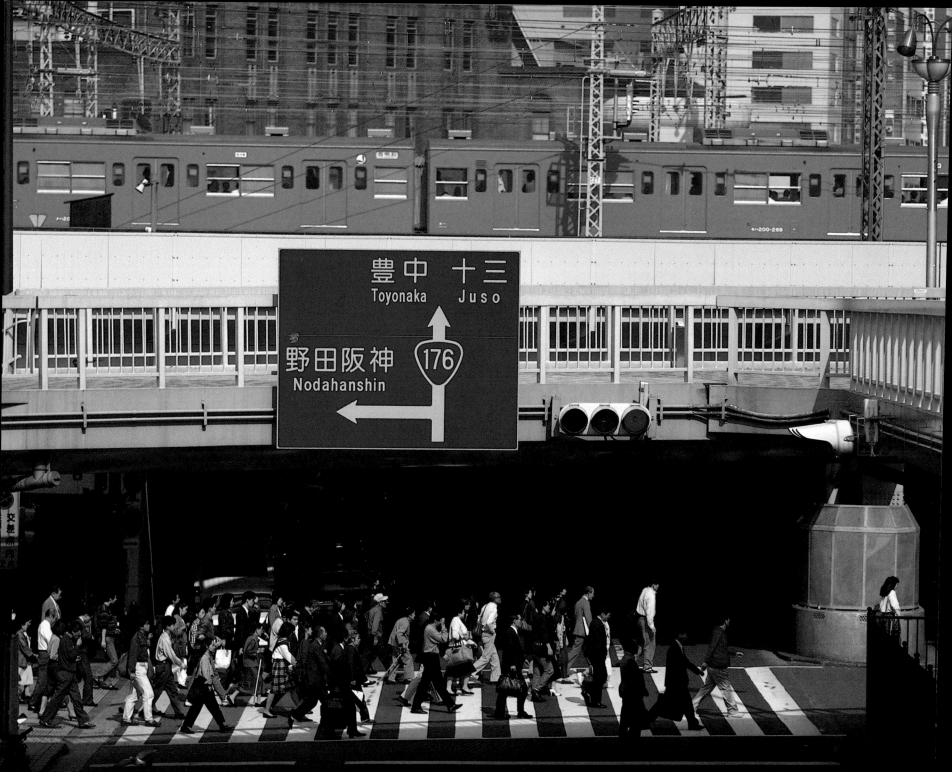

In India there were frequent complaints that the railways failed to provide food for third-class passengers. But this was a hopeless task since the country included people of two major religions, each with its own rules regulating the consumption of food, not to mention the Hindu caste system – which greatly complicated the task of the water carriers the companies provided. In particular high-caste Hindus needed reassurance that no member of certain inferior castes had touched their water, and would not fill their brass pots until they had conducted a lengthy interrogation on the subject.

In the United States the West (or rather the South West) was civilized by one Fred Harvey, who introduced fine dining halts the whole length of the Atchison Topeka and Santa Fe from Topeka to Los Angeles. Unfortunately, one habit he introduced, which has remained a feature of expensive American restaurants ever since, was not to use local produce, but to equate 'fine dining' with exotic food and wine.

That experienced traveller Paul Theroux even took the food as a gauge of a country's attitude towards its railways. In *The Old Patagonian Express*, he stated that they:

> ... told the whole story (and if there were no dining cars the country was beneath consideration). The noodle stall in the Malaysian train, the borscht and bad manners in the Trans-Siberian, the kippers and fried bread on the Flying Scotsman. And here on Amtrak's Lake Shore Limited I scrutinized the breakfast menu and discovered that it was possible for me to order a Bloody Mary or a Screwdriver ... There is not another train in the world where one can order a stiff drink at that hour of the morning. Amtrak was trying hard.

*B*ut the food served on the trains was the least of the services the railways performed to the world's dietary habits. At their most basic level, railways could prevent, or at least alleviate, famine. Most dramatically 'only' half a million Chinese died in a famine in 1920–1, whereas twenty-five times as many had died in a similar disaster which struck fifty years earlier, before the railways had reached the regions involved. Their vital role continues: the breakdown of the railways from the Indian Ocean to the interior has prevented aid from reaching the starving population of the southern Sudan over the past few years.

Opposite *The modern urban nightmare, Osaka-style.*

Railways were needed to prevent famines even in supposedly developed countries. As late as the 1840s much of rural France suffered from periodic food shortages, with their usual accompaniment of hoarding and profiteering. Within twenty years such dramas were forgotten, as were disparities in the prices of cereals – which in pre-railway days cost four times as much in the south of France as in the cereal-growing north.

Foodstuffs were not important only to the consumers, they were staple fare for the health of the railway companies themselves – in London and Paris a number of special stations were built to serve either individual markets, like the Smithfield meat market, or designed to deal with the hundreds of different products – most of them perishable – which poured into the metropolis every night.

The foods they introduced provided unprecedented variety for previously desperately restricted urban diets. The most spectacular case of dietary (and environmental) improvement came from London where cows had been housed in incredible numbers right up until the 1860s when the capital was struck by a cattle plague. An enterprising dairyman,

In 1924 Italian cheeses could get to Bishopsgate Goods Yard in the City of London by train faster than they can today.

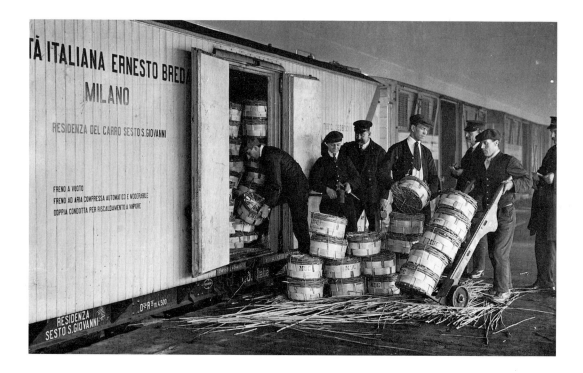

George Barham, rushed supplies of milk by train from outside London, and gave the company he founded a name emphasizing the speed with which the railways could bring fresh milk to his customers. Today Express Dairies still supplies fresh milk to more Londoners than any other company. Within a few years the milk traffic was so important that one of the GWR's routes in Wiltshire became known as the Milky Way.

The railways carried virtually every type of food and drink: there were banana (and coffee) railways throughout Central America, tea railways in Assam and Ceylon, and sugar lines in Cuba. Yet milk was the archetypal 'railway food' in that it was perishable and railways, as always, could transform the time required for a journey by fish or fruit or milk as much as by passengers.

Thanks to the railways (and to ice) fish was rushed overnight to London from Aberdeen, and villages in the west of Ireland could prosper because the mackerel caught by their fishermen could be on London's breakfast tables within twenty-four hours. For the benefits were not confined to the consumers – the railways transformed the prospects for peasants formerly obliged to sell to the nearest market-town. But the biggest benefit was for the urban poor. Radical historians have always insisted on the horrors of the earliest 'industrial' food, primitive margarine and mouldy corned beef: but railways made a triumphant exception. Only thanks to them did France's consumption of fruit and fresh vegetables double in the second half of the nineteenth century – at prices low enough to ensure that the proportion of the wage packet that went into food actually declined even as the variety available – and its quality – increased dramatically. Unfortunately one of the items whose price dropped most dramatically was the rough red wine the railways carried so cheaply from the South of France.

Almost as important was the railways' capacity to democratize foods which had previously been luxuries. The inhabitants of Zurich fondly called their first railway from Baden the Brötlibahn because it brought them their *brötli*, their favourite crisp breakfast rolls. Only trains could bring the early vegetables – the *primeurs* – so beloved of the Parisians from all over France to Paris, sea-food to land-locked Madrid or oysters the near-thousand miles from Baltimore Bay to Chicago. Because trains could extend the catchment area for urban markets the seasons during which city-dwellers could enjoy

Opposite *Vendors at Ollantaytambo station in Peru: the reality, as opposed to the ideal.*

An idealized vision of early railway travel in Japan by the artist Begg – note the shoes, which allegedly, passengers were apt to leave on the platform when embarking.

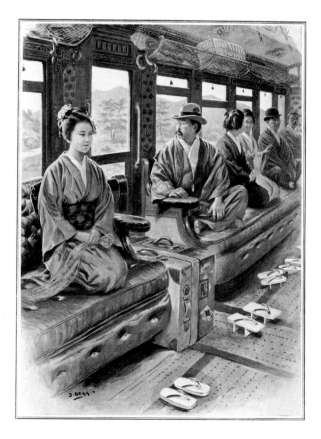

fresh fruit was greatly extended. Such traffic required vast quantities of ice, and in New England a whole new industry grew up to saw the ice from frozen ponds and transport it thousands of miles south to preserve fruit, fish, meat (and the ice-cold lager demanded by German immigrants).

The railways were not the first form of transport to democratize leisure. Before their arrival the steamship had transported thousands of holidaymakers on day trips down the Thames, or on longer journeys down the Mississippi and other major American waterways. But the railways were universal: they alone could provide holidaymakers with a choice of destinations. They enabled the inhabitants of the world's rapidly-growing cities to take advantage of their increasing but still minimal leisure time (in Britain Bank Holidays were introduced only in 1871). The railways also helped to expand and define the whole notion of the weekend. From the first they issued special tickets valid only over the weekend. The British gradually stopped working on Saturday afternoons, a practice followed slowly in continental Europe. And the whole mass of stories and legends attached to the country-house weekend favoured by the Edwardians depended on the trains which transported the guests (usually from Paddington) to the Cotswolds and to the mythical counties inhabited by the characters in the novels of P. G. Wodehouse.

The plebs had their place too in the railways' scheme of things. In Britain railways were used for excursion trains, either to the seaside – Brighton, Southend and Blackpool – or to Epping Forest and the banks of the Thames. These excursion trains – in the United States and France, as well as in Britain – were notoriously crowded. Then came more ambitious journeys, above all associated with the name of Thomas Cook. In 1841 he organized his first excursion train to transport a Temperance outing for a full 11 miles (18 kilometres). His biggest gamble came ten years later when he helped transport the masses of tourists who descended on London to visit the Great Exhibition. On one memorable day twenty special trains brought visitors to the metropolis.

Within a couple more decades Cook and his more business-like son had woven a dense network of tourist facilities throughout Europe and down into Egypt, held together

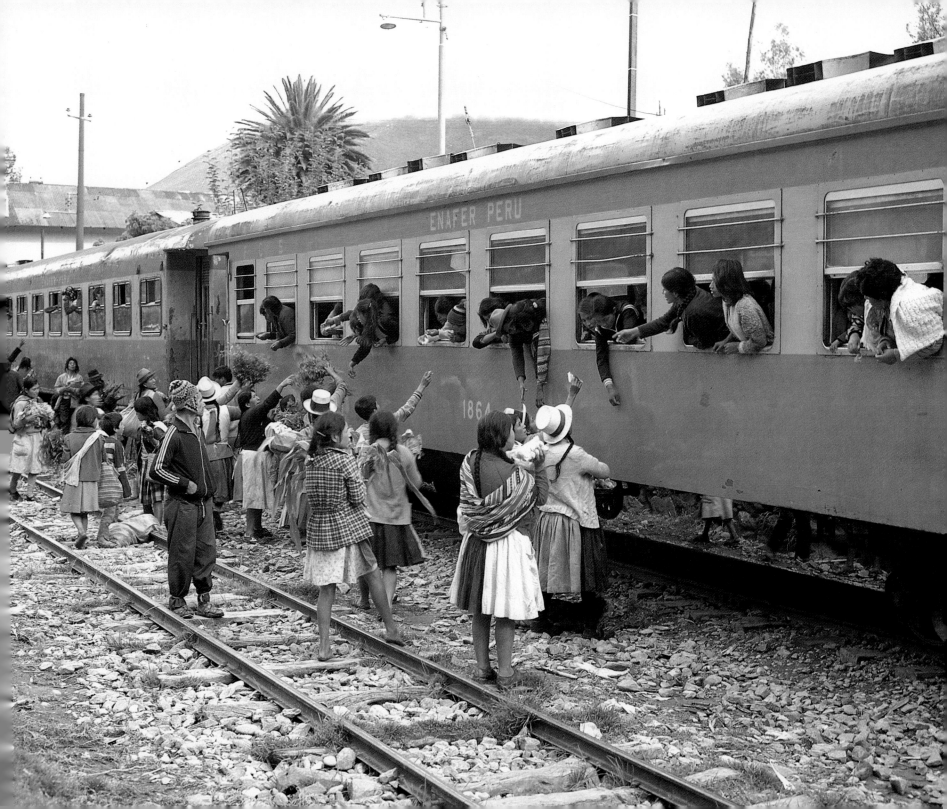

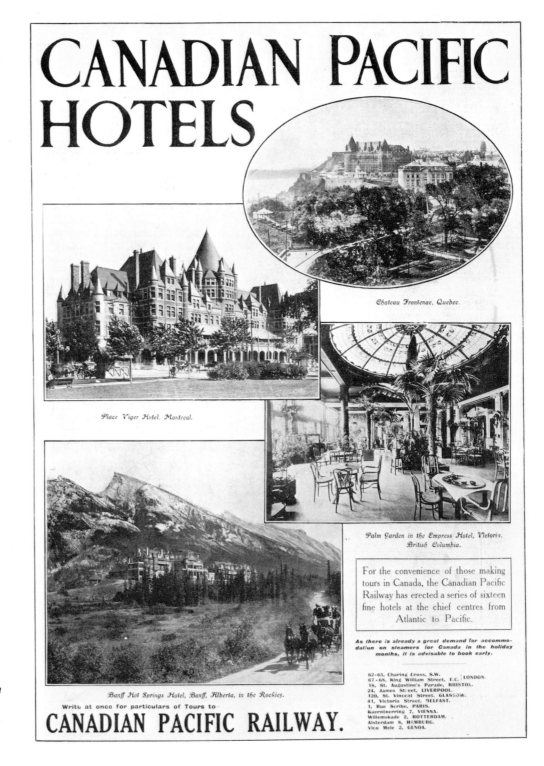

CANADIAN PACIFIC HOTELS

Chateau Frontenac, Quebec.

Place Viger Hotel, Montreal.

Palm Garden in the Empress Hotel, Victoria, British Columbia.

For the convenience of those making tours in Canada, the Canadian Pacific Railway has erected a series of sixteen fine hotels at the chief centres from Atlantic to Pacific.

As there is already a great demand for accommodation on steamers for Canada in the holiday months, it is advisable to book early.

62-65, Charing Cross, S.W.
67-68, King William Street, E.C. } LONDON.
18, St. Augustine's Parade, BRISTOL.
24, James Street, LIVERPOOL.
120, St. Vincent Street, GLASGOW.
41, Victoria Street, BELFAST.
1, Rue Scribe, PARIS.
Kaerntnerring 7, VIENNA.
Willemskade 2, ROTTERDAM.
Alsterdam 8, HAMBURG.
Vico Mele 2, GENOA.

Banff Hot Springs Hotel, Banff, Alberta, in the Rockies.

Write at once for particulars of Tours to

CANADIAN PACIFIC RAILWAY.

In Canada, as in Britain, the railways invented the whole idea of the 'resort hotel', many of them self-contained communities.

by the railways. There were regular trips to Switzerland – where Cook did more than the natives to develop skiing and mountaineering in the Alps – to Rome and Florence, and further afield. He even offered a journey to Turkey: 'With Constantinople for a centre', ran one brochure, 'may be visited the principal battlefields of the Russo-Turkish war, the Dardanelles, and the reputed site of Troy.' Cook not only created the traffic, he aroused the first complaints in a snobby line which has grown and flourished to this day: the groans, sometimes but not always justified, by those who feel that their best-loved retreats have been invaded and spoilt by hordes of tourists.

All this increased travelling inevitably led to the expansion of old-established resorts like Brighton or Saratoga Springs, the haunt of wealthy New Yorkers, and the creation of new ones. Many started as fishing villages, only to be transformed by the influx of tourists by rail – Cornwall with its colony of artists at St Ives being an obvious example. Such resorts did not have to be beside the seaside. Many, especially in continental Europe, formed a network of spas, like Carlsbad and Baden-Baden, where the rich and famous gathered every summer to reduce their waistlines (and to gossip). In India cool mountain resorts like Poona and Simla, the country's summer capital, fulfilled a similar function.

The railway companies went out of their way to encourage such traffic, often by building resort hotels. From their earliest days they had seen the attraction of including hotels in their plans for stations – the first was in Birmingham as early as 1839, a precedent followed by the builders of many of London's termini, like Victoria, Charing Cross, Paddington, King's Cross, and, most glamorously, St Pancras. But in a second phase the railway promoters realized that hotels could attract a new class of tourist, well-heeled, but without the social connections to enable them to stay with friends in the country. So they built 'golfers' hotels' like those at Turnberry near Ayr and Gleneagles, then as now a byword for luxury, built by the Caledonian Railway on its main line through Perthshire.

When Henry Flagler pushed his railway down the east coast of Florida he created some splendid resort hotels, including the Ponce de Leon in the old Spanish town of Saint Augustine and the Royal Ponciana, the biggest resort hotel in the world when it was built in the late 1890s, which promptly became a venue for some of the most

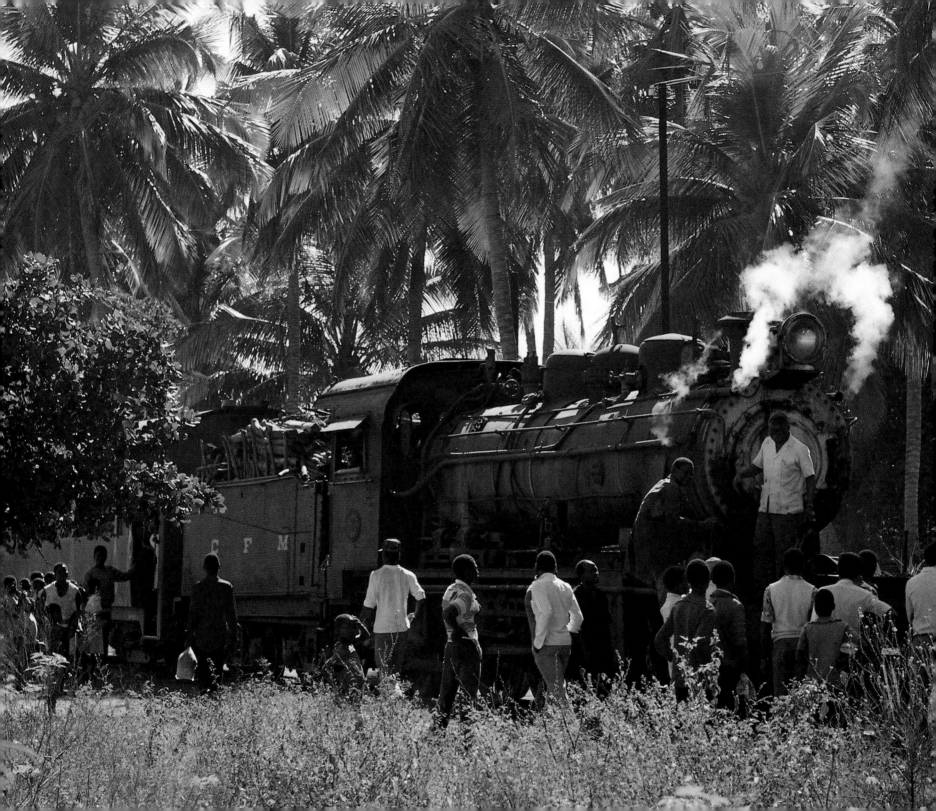

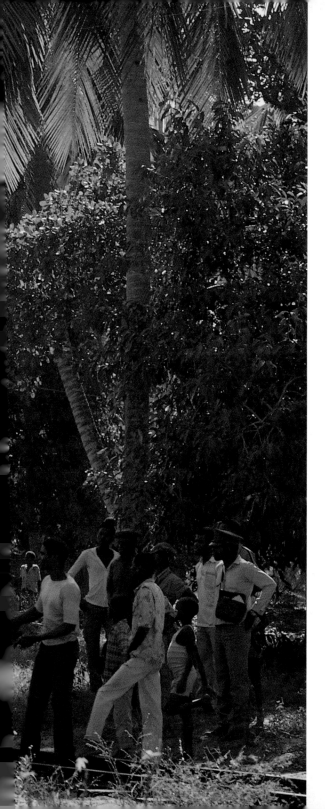

extravagant New Year's Eve parties of the Gilded Age. These places were more select than the future tourist monster he fathered from what had previously been merely a little fishing village at the mouth of the Miami River – a new town which the grateful natives wanted to call Flagler Beach.

His achievements had been foreshadowed on a smaller scale by two French bankers, the Pereire brothers. In the 1850s they built a line from Bordeaux to the little fishing port of Arcachon, previously inaccessible because of the surrounding marshes. As a result Arcachon became a fashionable resort – visitors included the composer Gounod who complained that he couldn't get away from his Parisian friends there. Many of the villas – built in their own very special style – were owned by the Chartronnais, the wealthy (mostly British) wine merchants from Bordeaux, who used to establish their families there for the whole summer, while the lower orders had to content themslves with Sunday excursions on trains of legendary discomfort.

But the railways' most glamorous creation was the French Riviera. A handful of wealthy British tourists had already discovered the little fishing village of Cannes before it was accessible by rail, but it and, especially, smaller settlements like Menton, were transformed into major resorts by the railway. A French hotelier, François Blanc, had an even more exciting vision: he foresaw the possible transformation of the impoverished principality of Monaco. Two previous operators of the casino had gone broke, but Blanc took a lease for a period which, he calculated quite rightly, would overlap with the arrival of the railway. The result: fame and fortune for him, and the emergence of Monte Carlo as the symbol of luxury and decadence in the second half of the nineteenth century, with Russian Grand Dukes jostling at the tables with the world's most beautiful, and best paid, *demi-mondaines* – not to mention The Man Who Broke The Bank at Monte Carlo.

A steam train in Mozambique. Picturesque, yes, but also crucial for the life of the country.

The railways' unequalled capacity to transport masses of people was put to its most severe test on the occasion of the major sporting events which it encouraged. All goods traffic was suspended the day the St Leger was run at Doncaster – not surprisingly since by 1888 the race they called 'the pitman's Derby' was attracting 100,000 racegoers brought in by excursion trains. Test matches also pulled crowds, and the railways put on additional excursion trains when the first Australian cricket team toured the country in 1878. But it was football, and above all the FA Cup Final, which stretched the railways' resources to the fullest.

The railways' 'discretionary' traffic, as opposed to passengers moving about their daily business by rail, was not only secular: an important proportion was bound on religious journeys. At first religious authorities were rather wary of the railways. There was rumbling discontent in both Britain and the United States over the desecration of the Sabbath by railways, which generally won the argument.

In Britain, however, there has always been an empathy between trains and the Church of England, generally more tolerant of Sabbath-breaking than more Puritan sects. Ecclesiastical and railway history is full of stories of clergymen – most obviously the great Archbishop William Temple – who knew Bradshaw, the complete railway timetable, by heart, and it seemed natural that the adventures of Thomas The Tank Engine and his friends should be recounted by a clergyman – the Reverend Wilbert Awdry.

The most famous ecclesiastical objection to trains was by the Orthodox Russian bishops, worried at the construction of a railway to the Troitsk monastery: '. . . In railway cars . . . all sorts of tales can be heard, and often dirty stories, whereas now they come on foot and each step is a feat pleasing to God.' But they soon relented and within a few years religious authorities the world over were providing railway builders with some of their best opportunities. In Japan, for example, several lines were built specially to serve shrines. The first railway in what was then Persia was to connect Tehran with a nearby shrine, and in India the railways spurred on an enormous growth in the numbers going on pilgrimages. This traffic was considered so important that Robert Stephenson consulted 'the great Sanhedrin of orthodox Hindoos' before going ahead with one new line (fortunately the Sanhedrin duly gave its blessing). The most spectacular use of railways to democratize pilgrimages and thus provide a boost to the religions involved were Catholic and Muslim. Only trains enabled unprecedented masses of pilgrims to reach Lourdes and later Mecca.

From the railways' point of view Bernadette Soubirous' visions could not have been better timed. She saw them just as the (Jewish) Pereires were deciding the route of their railway line south of Bordeaux, and the local council of Lourdes ensured that it passed through the town. By 1866, a mere eight years after her first visions, the little town was directly linked with Bordeaux, 200 miles (322 km) to the north, and even with Paris. As a result over 650,000 pilgrims flocked to Lourdes in the eight years between 1870 and 1878, and 100,000 came on a single day to rejoice in the newly established doctrine of the Immaculate Conception.

In France the use of railways was further institutionalized by the Assumptionists, a mass religious movement with rather sinister right-wing political overtones which systematically used special trains to assemble the faithful for the mass rallies which formed an important part of its strategy.

In France the faithful did not have to build their own railways. In the Ottoman Empire they did. In 1900 Sultan Abdul Hamid proposed to build a railway to Mecca as a pious gesture to mark the twenty-fifth anniversary of his accession to the throne. A combination of piety, unlimited resources and the genius of the German engineer, Meissner Pasha, ensured that within eight years 1600 km (1000 miles) of railway line was built, mostly through trackless desert, and the line reached Medina in 1908. But it was used only for eight years until T. E. Lawrence blew it up in an explosion which every film-goer can recall, since when the track has lain rusting in the desert, its neglect a tribute to the consequences of the break-up of the Ottoman empire (and, more recently, to the rise of air travel).

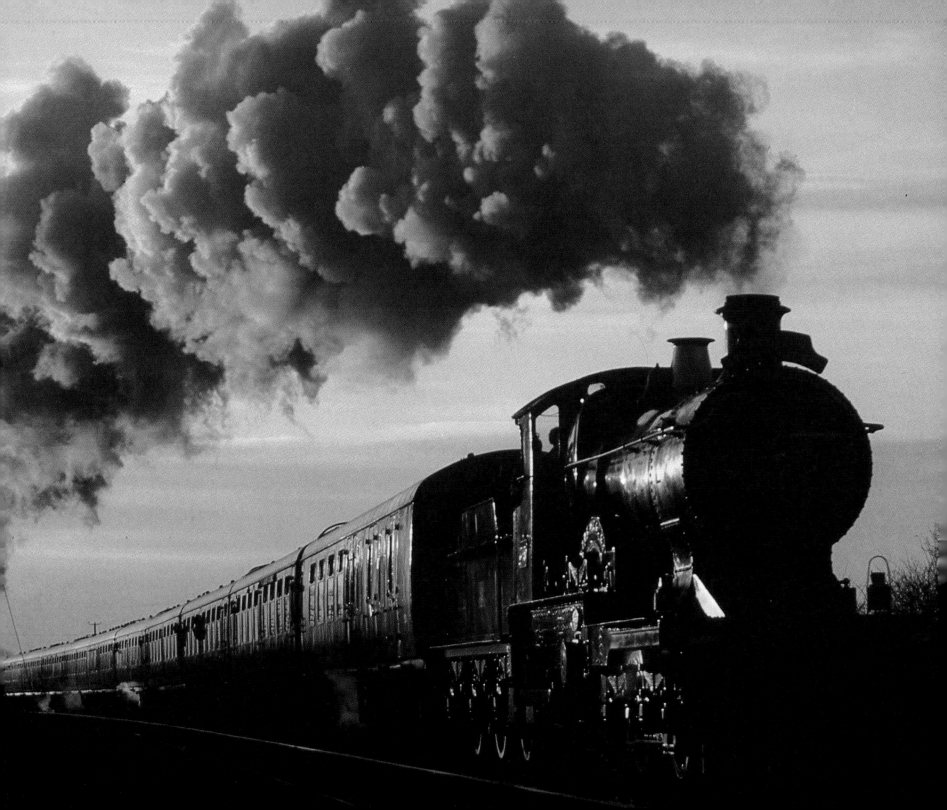

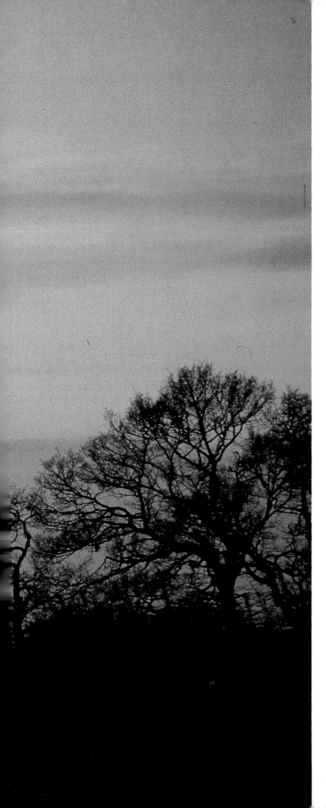

8　Temples of Steam

Railways were the biggest infrastructure projects undertaken since Roman times. Before the arrival of motorways (at a time of far greater technological sophistication, when machines had largely replaced human muscle power) they remained miracles of construction the world over. Only the railway builders could cross rivers and deserts, only they could tunnel under mountains which previous generations had neither the will nor the finance to conquer. And because railways were the dominant industrial and financial force for so much of the nineteenth century, the buildings associated with them were the single most important and widespread form in which contemporary architecture expressed itself. Railway lines, bridges and viaducts were the natural outlets for the talents of engineering geniuses like Brunel and Eiffel. The trains, the locomotives and the carriages which ran over their lines were equally unforgettable.

Yet, for all the magnificence of the buildings for which they were responsible, railway companies started by acting as unimaginably violent agents of destruction, most memorably described by Charles Dickens in *Dombey and Son*:

> The first shock of a great earthquake had, just at that period, rent the whole neighbourhood to its centre. Traces of its course were visible on every side. Houses were knocked down; streets broken through and stopped; deep pits and trenches dug in the ground; enormous heaps of earth and clay thrown up; buildings that were undermined and shaking, propped by great beams of wood. Here, a chaos of carts, overthrown and jumbled together, lay topsy-

The City of Truro, the first locomotive to break the 100 mph barrier in Britain – naturally on Brunel's Great Western Railway.

165

turvy at the bottom of a steep unnatural hill; there, confused treasures of iron soaked and rusted in something that had accidentally become a pond.

The most original structures were the lines themselves and the bridges and viaducts associated with them, virtually all still in use, and the tunnels, each with its own tragic story to tell. From the beginning every one, seemingly, set some sort of record: in Britain the longest tunnel, first at Kilsby between London and Birmingham, then at Box between London and Bristol, was soon followed by the horrors associated with the building of the Woodhead Tunnel under the Pennines. A couple of decades later the Severn Tunnel was the longest in the world at the time, and the builders had to cope with a tidal wave as well as problems with unexpected geological faults.

British authors naturally concentrate on these, the early, domestic conquests of nature, and tend to overlook the generally far greater and more difficult triumphs over nature involved in tunnelling under the Apennines, conquered by Germain Someiller, the inventor of the pneumatic drill, and the Alps. The St Gotthard, most crucial of tunnels since it was the key point on the historic route between northern and southern Europe, was the scene of numerous tragedies and the deaths of many of the leading figures involved in its construction, including Alfred Escher, the tunnel's promoter, and Louis Favre, the Genevan contractor who died bankrupt and was buried alongside hundreds of the tunnel's other victims.

Inevitably projects outside Europe became tests of the technical skills of the major manufacturing countries, and foreshadowed the American technological supremacy which was to be so notable a feature of the history of the twentieth century.

American bridge engineering triumphed in Burma, where the fabled Goktiek Bridge was transported in sections all the way from Pennsylvania, and in the Andes, where they built the Verrugas Bridge at an altitude of 1800 m (6000 ft) over a tributary of the Rimac, an achievement worthily celebrated in a medal made by Louis Tiffany. The French had used their own men to launch already prefabricated structures, an approach which proved a failure. The Americans erected a bridge weighing 81 tonnes in eight days, while the comparable British-built structure weighed twice as much and would have taken twice as long to put up.

The obstacles overcome included a vertical mountain wall impossible to tunnel through – for which the contractor, Henry Meiggs, invented the 'Meiggs v-switch' to enable the line to corkscrew its way up the steepest of slopes. Another was used in a tunnel further up a track which ended at over 4600 m (15,000 ft), above the summit of Mont Blanc, Europe's highest mountain. The railway also traversed a ledge with a 600 m (2000 ft) perpendicular wall on one side and an even deeper vertical drop on the other, and tunnels containing galleries of tracks one above another.

Railway miracles were required even over flat and apparently peaceful terrain. As G. W. MacGeorge wrote in his book *Ways and Works in India*, at least one stretch of the railway from Calcutta to Delhi:

> ... traverses a low portion of deltaic land, subject to extreme inundation for the water system
> of the country ... over this wide expanse of level country, subject to an excessive tropical
> rainfall, inundations from the flood spill of the enormous channel of the Ganga and other
> great rivers are often spread as a vast sheet over miles of country, converting the whole
> district into the semblance of an inland sea.

At first the railway, like the modern motorway, seemed an appalling intrusion into the landscape, for earlier roads, and indeed canals, had followed the lines of a landscape, not imposed themselves on it. Inevitably John Ruskin, the enemy of industrialization in all its forms, saw in the railway the perfect symbol of all he hated, and his fulminations (like Fanny Kemble's eulogy) remain the standard point of reference for railway historians. In *Praeterita* he thundered how:

> ... you enterprised a railway through a valley, you blasted its rocks away, heaped thousands
> of tons of shale into its lovely stream. The valley is gone, and the Gods with it; and every
> fool in Buxton can be in Bakewell in half an hour, and every fool in Bakewell in Buxton;
> which you think a lucrative process of exchange, you Fools everywhere.

But it was William Wordsworth who earned further immortality as the first Nimby, the first prominent person to object to a railway In his Back Yard. A proposed line to Lake Windermere triggered the famous sonnet: 'Is there no nook of English ground secure from rash assault?' which he combined with a spate of exceptionally snobby

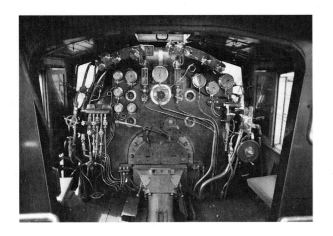

The gleaming glory of the cab on a steam locomotive: a tradition maintained in South Africa if nowhere else.

letters to the *Morning Post* (in the end it was financial problems, rather than the poet's objections, which stopped the line).

By the time the motor car arrived the railway line, especially through rural areas, had become an accepted part of the scenery, its natural relationship with the landscape if anything enhanced by wisps of steam from the engines. And most modern observers would agree with Moray Maclaren's description of the Highland Railway, which, he wrote (in *Return to Scotland*):

> ... does not rob anything of the grandeur from the scenery through which it passes. It is so insignificant, its trains pass so seldom and so slowly, it no more takes away the desolation from the Highlands for the traveller than does the sight of an Atlantic liner minimise for the swimmer the vastness of the ocean. Roads can much more effectively destroy this quality.

The lines were only part of the total railway phenomenon. The locomotives themselves were the symbols of the railway revolution for a variety of reasons: because they were handsome objects, because of the noise, the orgasmic grunts which accompanied their departure, the clouds of steam which so mysteriously enveloped them. Poets could use them to express their feelings, but most of the fictional portrayals harked back to the theme, first stated by Fanny Kemble, of the locomotive, metaphorically as well as literally, as an Iron Horse. Emily Dickinson saw the locomotive as a friendly, domesticated beast which, after demonstrating almost supernatural powers over nature would:

> *Stop – docile and omnipotent –*
> *At its own stable door.*

Earlier, Walt Whitman had found his own reasons, which come down to sex and power, to worship the locomotive beast, with its '... *train of cars ... thy swinging lamps at night ... thy fierce-throated beauty ... in thy panoply, thy measur'd dual throbbing and thy beat convulsive.*'

*T*he chief glory of the railways has always been their stations. All the greatest architects of the nineteenth and early twentieth century were naturally employed to design them, for the very simple reason that they were the biggest and most prestigious commissions on offer. The railways were sometimes directly connected with other major buildings, as exemplified by the story of the Crystal Palace, which housed the Great Exhibition of 1851. The project depended on the financial impetus provided by Sir Samuel Morton Peto, the railway entrepreneur, and the revolutionary design of its spectacular glass structure was approved by Robert Stephenson and supervised by Mr Barlow, the 'eminent engineer' of the Midland Railway. Its design was then used as the pattern for a number of great steam train sheds, like that at London's St Pancras Station.

But train sheds did not a station make. Station buildings were not often original, they simply expressed the railways' role as mirrors of society. The promoters, like all *nouveaux riches* throughout the ages, preferred to stick to existing forms, merely showing off by using these forms in an extravagant fashion. They wanted to impress, and the way they knew best was to outdo rivals, but not to shock them. As a result they did not innovate, but echoed contemporary styles, even, indeed especially, when they were at their most extravagant. Nevertheless nineteenth-century stations remained the supreme symbols of the triumph of the railways, their owners, and the powers behind them. It was only a later generation which used railway stations to express new ideas – like Eero Saarinen's station in Helsinki, built in 1910, and the famous terminus in Rome built after the Second World War.

The desire to fit in was perfectly natural. Railways were a dangerous novelty, and their promoters were naturally anxious to reassure travellers that the buildings, at least, were of familiar design and shape, reminiscent of other public buildings, like town halls and museums.

The very first proper station set the pattern. At Crown Street in Liverpool the passenger arrived at a vehicle court and found himself in a room used both as a ticket office and a waiting room. The architect – or rather the unknown builders and engineers working for George Stephenson – simply solved the technical problems posed by the passengers' needs within the framework of the contemporary vernacular.

Within a few years architects showed how well they could adapt fashionable styles for railway-connected purposes, on the grandest of scales. The first major such example was Euston station, built at the end of the 1830s to house the London terminus of the railway from London to Birmingham, the first line between a country's two major cities.

Overleaf left Grand Central Station, New York, *one of the last of the great railway cathedrals – but not a 'Temple of Steam' because it was designed to be used only by electric locomotives.*

Overleaf right Lenin still looks down on waiting *passengers at Kiev station.*

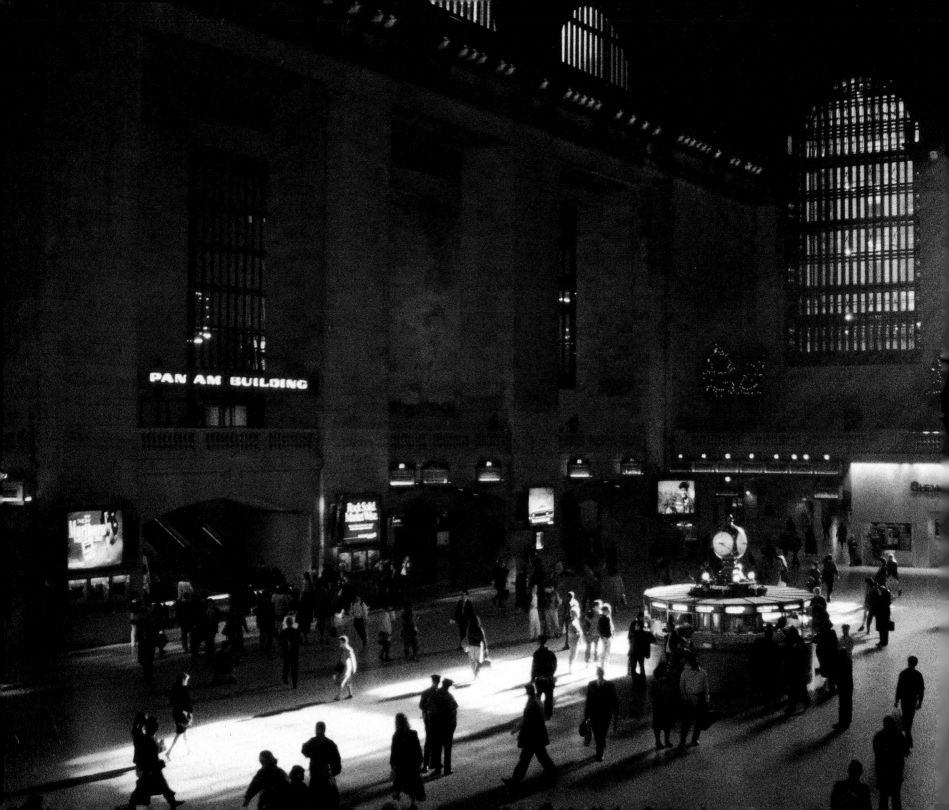

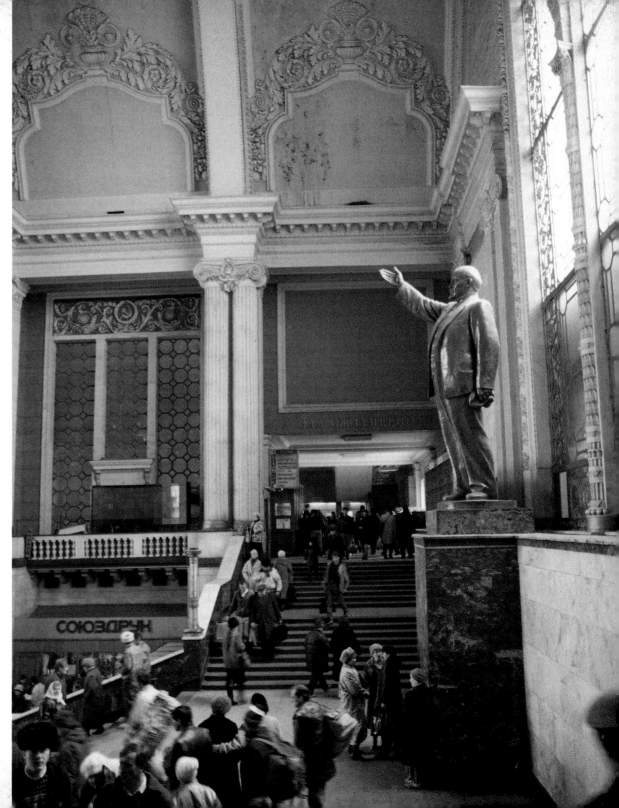

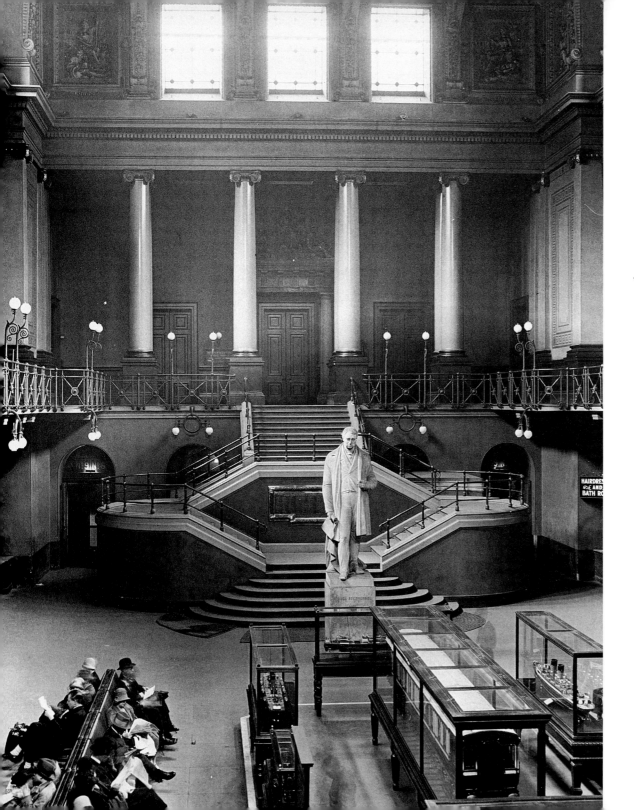

The first great Temple of Steam: the Great Hall at Euston Station, terminus for the London & Birmingham line. The statue is of Robert Stephenson, who built the line.

It included a triumphal arch, a hotel, a magnificent Great Hall and an equally splendid boardroom for the London and North Western. The approach was deliberate. As Gordon Biddle wrote (in *Great Railway Stations of Britain*): 'The whole purpose of the façade was to create a symbolic gateway to the railway, using the Roman triumphal arch as its theme', in line with the contemporary notion that classical antiquity was the model for all nobility, in architecture as in every other sphere of human activity. In the words of Nikolaus Pevsner, the 'styles were chosen for what they would evoke.'

To break with the classical models required courage. Only Brunel showed any real architectural originality to match the daring of the whole idea of steam-powered travel. Few stations were as architecturally original, or as integrated, as Paddington, where, in the words of Christian Barman in *An Introduction to Railway Architecture*: 'The whole of the train hall structure is treated as a single design ... in line with Brunel's invariable policy of designing everything from first principles, without regard to existing criteria.' One of the few other major stations where the style is as integrated is at Atocha in Madrid.

Ten years later at King's Cross the world saw the first Brutalist railway station, an unornamented engineering triumph, its purpose plain to see. But in London, as elsewhere in Europe, the characteristic pattern of the last quarter of the nineteenth century was for the two constructs – the train hall and the offices and façade – to be stylistically separate.

The 'normal' contrast is best summed up by St Pancras, King's Cross's neighbour, which showed the disintegration of the dream of a stylistically uniform railway station to the full. The train shed is itself a splendidly simple glass arch, at the time the widest single-span glass structure in the world. But its glory is hidden from the street by the complex façade, which contained a hotel as well as the station offices.

The building was originally planned – by Sir Giles Gilbert Scott, the most fashionable architect of the mid-Victorian era – to house Britain's Foreign Office. But the Foreign Secretary, Lord Palmerston, rejected the design and Scott persuaded the directors of the Midland Railway, clearly a body of men anxious to make a splash, to use it. It soon became mocked for its pretentiousness, but remains one of the best-loved features of London's skyline.

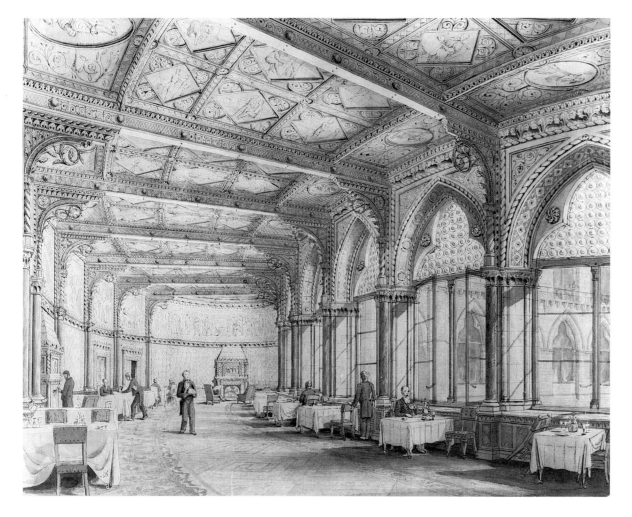

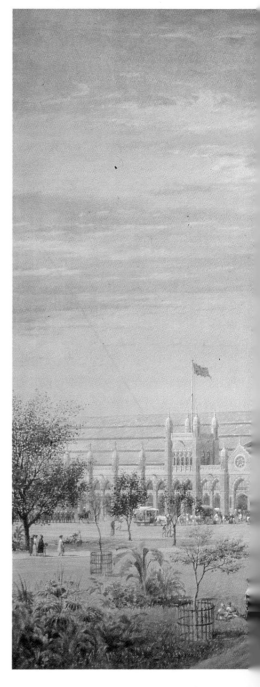

The Dining-Room at the St Pancras Hotel
in London, as envisaged by Sir Giles Gilbert Scott.

Right *Victoria Station Bombay, the ultimate in*
Imperial grandeur dreamed up by Axel Hermann Haig.

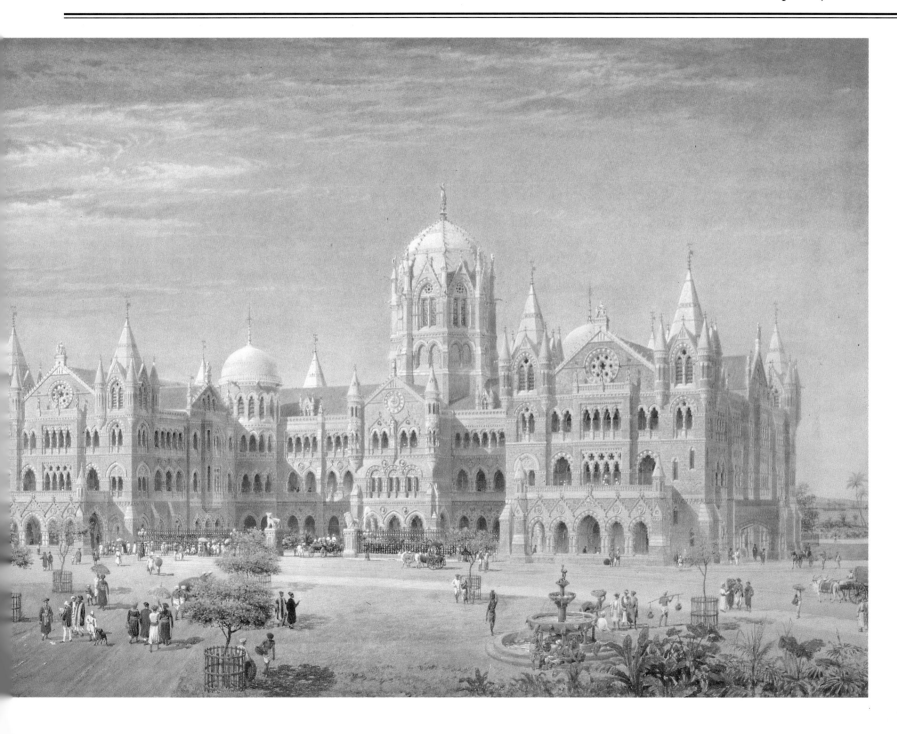

Unlike their successors, the world's airports, stations never developed an 'international style', but remained true to their origins. These were not necessarily national (there were quite a few 'imperial' stations) but they reflected the culture of the country or region involved. Atocha station in Madrid is recognizably Spanish, but its equivalent in Seville reflects the Moorish influence which remains so important throughout the south of Spain.

Outside major cities stations often showed the national dream at its purest. Rural England is littered with stations which resemble nothing so much as glorified cottages. In Switzerland and much of Scandinavia you find delightful chalets fulfilling the same purpose. But it is France, with its proud provincial tradition, where you find the greatest variety. At Vitré the station is a model chateau, complete with crenellations, and at Passy in Paris a charming classical cottage. The tradition continued between the wars. Caen provides a fine example of a sympathetically modernist structure, while the station at Hendaye, on the Spanish frontier, marries the two cultures.

In the United States the railway station had at first been a casual affair. According to Alvin E. Harlow, in *A Treasury of Railroad Folklore*:

> In the smaller towns, the railroad's representative was often the nearest storekeeper, and passengers had to await the trains in the store and buy tickets there too ... towns large enough to be called cities had real depots, barnlike structures through which the track or tracks ran as through a tunnel. Seats and a ticket office were close along the track. For winter days, huge swinging doors closed the openings at each end of the depot, though plenty of cold wind wailed under and around them for the discomfort of the passengers shivering in the seats, awaiting a train which might be delayed from half an hour to half a day – one never knew what to expect, because there was no telegraph to report its progress.

But within a few decades these unwelcoming barns had become the social centre of many small towns, and the pride and joy of most American cities, the very symbol of the unity for which the nation was striving after the Civil War. Most major cities had their, usually classical, always impressive, Union Station. And suitably, one of the finest was in Washington, where it is strategically placed at one corner of the hill which houses so many of the nation's other major federal institutions, including Congress.

For railway stations were important symbols of a country's (or its ruler's) perception of itself. This could be muddled. In India three markedly different stations each symbolize one element in British rule. The enormous Victoria Terminus in Bombay is an unhappy attempt to reinterpret indigenous Indian architectural styles and translate them into modern (i.e. Victorian) terms. The result is a nightmare which makes St Pancras seem positively restrained. At Lahore the defensive element is emphasized: the station is designed like a fort. At Delhi, a proposed station, like so much else in the city, was designed to emphasize the glory of Britain's imperial rule.

The same imperialist triumphalism was expressed with greater brutality and vulgarity at Metz, one of the cities annexed by the Germans after the Franco-Prussian war of 1870. They celebrated their victory by constructing a vast, incongruous castle of a station which could never have been designed by a Frenchman. Elsewhere the connotations surrounding stations could be sombre, because they were associated with wartime farewells. In London most termini witnessed sentimental scenes as evacuees were despatched to the country at the outbreak of the Second World War, and Waterloo carries a memorial plaque to the hundreds of thousands of servicemen who passed through on their way to the front in the First World War. In Paris the Gare de L'Est has its own memorial, a mural commemorating that fact that it served the same purpose on at least three occasions – in 1870, 1914 and 1939. Not surprisingly the streets round the station are named after major battles.

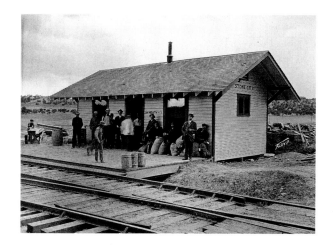

The station at Stone City, one of a thousand such lonely and anonymous outposts.

A city's major station was naturally perceived as second only to its town hall in symbolic and practical significance. This increased the pressure on the railway companies. In Amsterdam, typically, the burghers insisted that the city's gigantic station should be situated outside its historic heart, and that it should be designed in a style in keeping with the rest of the city. The result may dominate its surroundings, but only through its sheer bulk, not through any stylistic incongruity.

Railway stations often created their own buzz, their own ferment of development. This was partly because, in large cities like London, the first termini had to be on the outskirts – as were Paddington and the three northern termini, Euston, King's Cross and

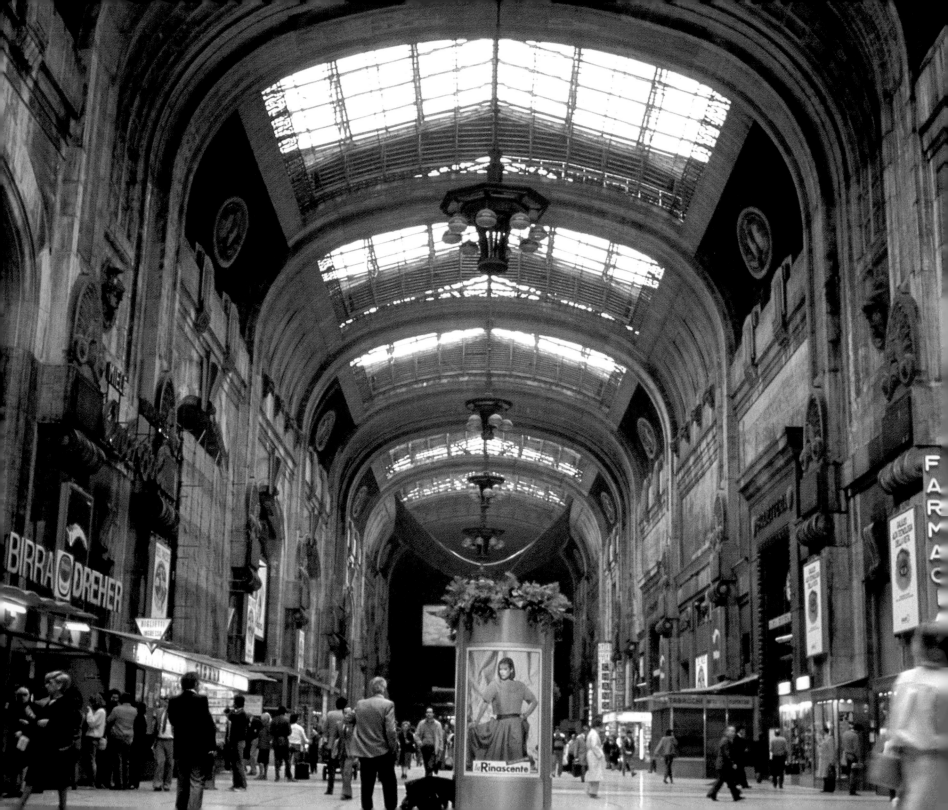

St Pancras, at the time they were built. But none of the new 'railway quarters' were at all appetizing: stations like Paddington and King's Cross in London and the Gare de Lyon and the Gare St Lazare in Paris are still surrounded by a mass of sleazy hotels, and the roads round about are still crowded with prostitutes. Even in well-ordered Zurich, although the road leading to the station (the Bahnhofstrasse, famous for its bankers) is an elegant boulevard, the surroundings of the station itself were never very stylish or impressive.

There were exceptions. In Liverpool the City Council insisted that the station should fit in with its greatest secular building, St George's Hall, and in Paris Haussmann placed the grandiose Gare de l'Est as the culminating point of one of his most important new boulevards. In the words of Wolfgang Schievelbusch (in *The Railway Journey*), he built the Boulevard de Strasbourg as a:

> ... direct continuation of the rails, mathematically parallel and just as linear. Like the railway line in open terrain, the boulevard struck across the cityscape, cutting heedlessly through whatever was in its way ... even Haussmann's other main thoroughfares can be perceived as complements to rail traffic. They either connect the terminals with the centre of the city or with each other.

Only late in the nineteenth century did stations start to form an integral part of a new quarter worthy of their own grandeur. In Europe the best examples are in Antwerp and Milan. In Antwerp the result was a triumph celebrating the arts and crafts movement of the period, whereas in Milan the façade, at least, is Babylonian-Fascist (it was only finished in Mussolini's time, in 1931) although the interior conforms to our ideas of nineteenth-century Italian urban design, with elegant gallerias and expansive public spaces.

Tracks and stations could be terribly intrusive. You have only to go to Southwark in London to see how the railway, in penetrating into the heart of the city, destroyed the surroundings of one of Britain's finest smaller cathedrals. Many an American town was bisected by railway tracks, but these usually belonged to the railroad to which the community involved owed its very existence, and did not crash through an existing settlement.

Opposite *The Galleria at Milan's central station, an elegant nineteenth century addition to the city's facilities.*

179

Brussels is the only city of any size whose historic heart was ripped asunder and permanently scarred by the railway – an object lesson unfortunately not learnt by builders of urban motorways a generation later. For over half a century development through a swathe of the city was frozen to preserve the railways' route connecting the city's two existing (and perfectly adequate) termini. All this was the result of a bizarre obsession: never mind that cities like London, Paris and Berlin did not have trains running through their heart, Brussels had to offer passengers a through route.

Of course there were many instances of vandalism as the railways crashed into the heart of other cities, but these generally concerned individual buildings. In Liverpool and Edinburgh medieval churches were pulled down; in York a section of the Roman wall was sacrificed; and in Cologne installation of a railway station in the crowded old town involved the destruction of the city's only green space, its botanical garden. For the construction of an impressive station was considered worth a sacrifice or a lengthy battle: indeed Limoges struggled for three-quarters of a century before a station worthy of the city was finally completed, as late as 1929.

In New York, as in London and Paris, the tracks were not, initially, allowed to penetrate into the heart of the city. But at the turn of the century two great termini, Penn Station at 34th Street and, above all, Grand Central eight blocks further north, helped inspire the move of the city's commercial heart uptown to what is now 'midtown' and remains at the heart of the city's life. By contrast, British stations were not generally social focal points, though there was one exception, the Central Station in Glasgow, a 'treasured possession of the city' in Jack Simmons' words, which 'afforded hospitality to many thousands of people who were not passengers.'

Grand Central, like the Gare d'Orsay in Paris, was designed to be used only by electric locomotives, which gave the designers far more freedom – notably that they didn't have to leave open ends or a well-ventilated roof to allow the smoke to escape. Grand Central was itself imposing. Indeed the *New York Times* considered it as 'a gateway to the nation and – for inbound passengers – to the city.' It was also the model of the future city, not the city beautiful (though its Romanesque architecture delighted reviewers) but the city efficient. For with Grand Central the station started to become not a symbol of the power of the company that had built it or the city to which it was the 'entrance', but part of the social engineering of urban life and an affirmation of effective management.

*D*uring the railways' first surge, they did not generally depend on commuters – indeed many major railways, like the Great Western, rather discouraged them, preferring freight and longer-distance travellers. Even in the 1860s, when much of the rail network to London was complete, only one in ten of London's 600,000 commuters travelled by train and in the United States most urban centres remained 'walking cities', their further spread usually delayed until the arrival of the motor car.

The first 'Tube', from Paddington to the City of London, opened in 1863, was not primarily to serve commuters, but inhabitants of inner London working in the city. Indeed, because in Britain at least, the railways themselves were not legally allowed to indulge in property development, urban railways tended to follow existing patterns of settlement, not create new suburbs. In London the major exception was the Metropolitan Railway, which between the wars created what was fondly known as Metroland, the once much derided but extremely agreeable band of newly built suburbs which stretched out beyond the existing bounds of north-west London.

Urban railways, like national ones, echoed national aspirations, national habits. The 'metros' in New York and London grew haphazardly; that in Paris was a later, more consciously planned development – and Glasgow's position in the late nineteenth century as the world's leading engineering centre was symbolized by the fact that it possessed one of the world's first urban railway systems.

During the 1930s thousands of Russian labourers worked themselves to death under the command of a young thug called Nikita Krushchev to provide Moscow with a splendid underground system which would be a witness to the progress the country had made under Stalin. During the excavations the workers came across a sinister and symbolic relic: a courtyard used by Ivan the Terrible to house his prisoners, whose torture became a spectator sport for him. But then the whole project resembled more the construction of the pyramids, a tribute to the glory of a primitive tyrant, rather than a mundane attempt to provide better transportation.

Shimbashi station in the heart of Tokyo as seen by the artist Kiyochika.

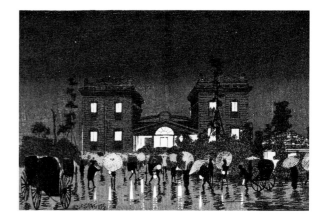

Both the Paris and the Moscow systems were completed in great haste for prestige purposes, in Paris to cope with the hordes of visitors expected for the 1900 Universal Exhibition and in Moscow to celebrate the seventeenth anniversary of the Revolution on 7 November 1934.

The Paris system was the result of a typical political battle between the French state and the city, which had been deprived of its independence as a result of the revolt of the Commune in 1871. In the event the city tricked the state by ensuring that the tunnels were too narrow to use main-line rolling stock. But then the relationship between metropolitan railways and commuter lines has always been tricky. For decades London Transport and British Rail could not agree to provide a single ticket serving both systems, and only recently (most obviously in Germany) have cities managed to integrate the two, a process which has now spread to such major British conurbations as Manchester with its Metrorail system.

But however forward-looking the network, the construction of an underground system merely put off the evil day when gridlock would prevail. This was foreseen by William Barclay Parsons, engineer of the first New York Subway. Just two months after the opening ceremony he wrote how property owners were already planning to build along the whole line. As a result:

> By the time the railway is completed, areas that are now given over to rocks and goats will be covered with houses, and there will be created for each new line, just as there has been created for each new line constructed in the past, a special traffic of its own, independent of the normal growth of the city. The instant that this line is finished there will arise a demand for other lines.

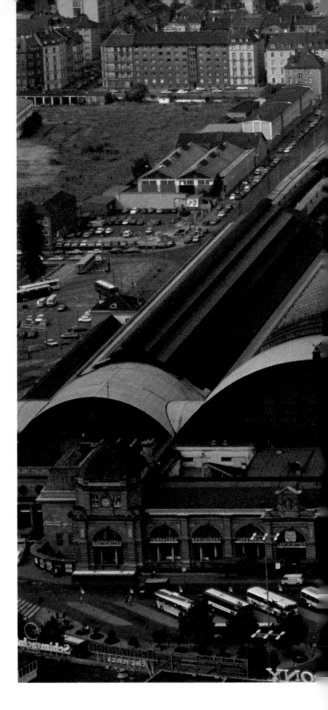

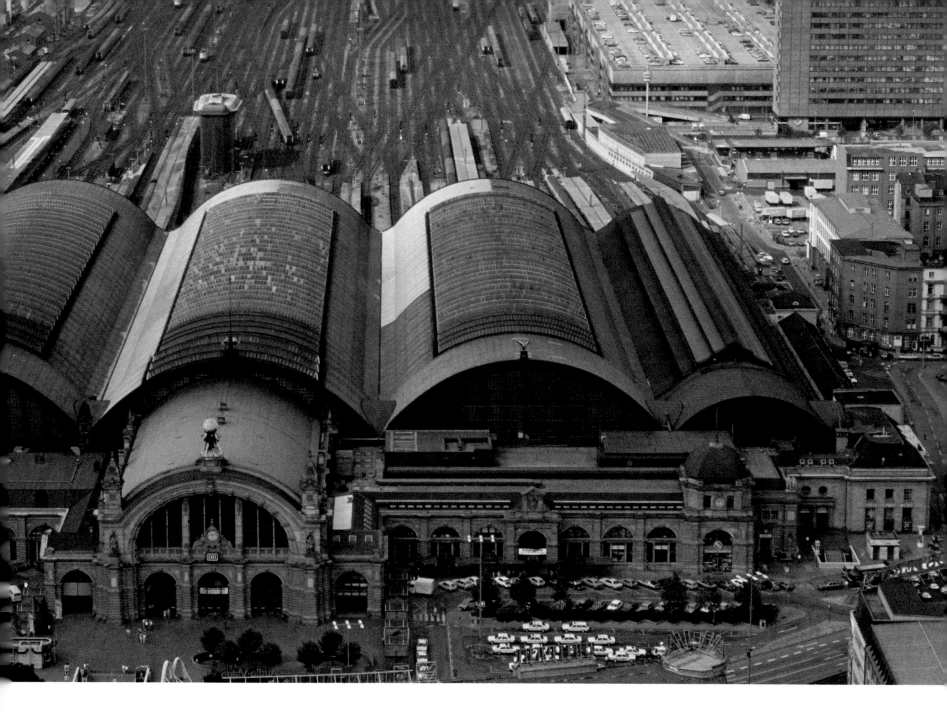

*The Station at Frankfurt am Main, one of the many such monsters built by
competitive German cities in the last quarter of the nineteenth century.*

9 *Railway Art*

Steam engines, trains, stations, were all gifts to novelists, artists and, in the twentieth century, to film-makers. The railways touched every aspect of creative art one way or another, as an inspiration, or simply as a means of spreading an art-form or popular amusement.

The most obvious type of entertainment which owes everything to the railways' carrying capacity is the circus, which needed special trains to move its elaborate equipment and hordes of animals. The modern circus was created, not, as people tend to assume, by the great showman P. T. Barnum, but by a much less well-known figure, one William Cameron Coup. He organized circuses mounted on standard flat cars which could travel a hundred miles overnight and still perform the next day; he even had special trains sent in advance with agents arousing excitement with the promise that 'the circus is coming to town' and drumming up advance ticket sales.

The railways could themselves provide raw material. The public, then as now, loved the sheer horror and drama of crashes. Best-selling prints and ballads about railways usually involved crashes, though not, curiously, the biggest ones – apart from a few spectaculars, like the collapse of the Tay Bridge. It was the fate of individuals, most notably Casey Jones, which particularly intrigued the public. By a natural extension a character appropriately named 'Head-on' Joe Connolly earned a handsome living for over thirty years by staging crashes all over the United States. He would buy a couple of clapped-out locomotives, lay over half a mile of track at the spacious grounds where State Fairs were held, hire skilled (and nerveless) engineers and wait for the thousands of punters prepared to pay for the result. In all Joe staged seventy-five head-on collisions, and could boast that no one had been hurt, let alone killed, in any of them.

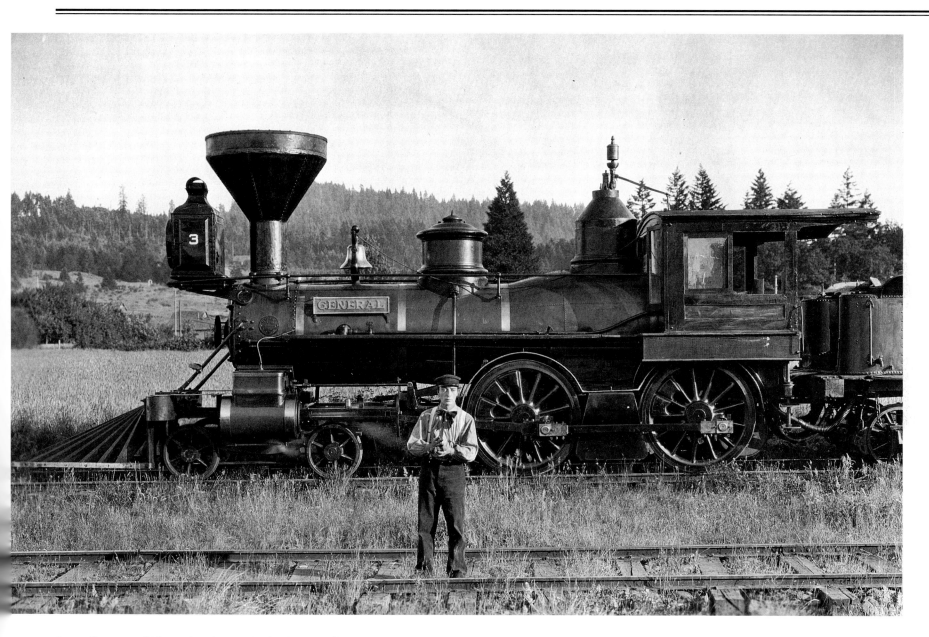

Buster Keaton and his precious locomotive in the 1927 film The General, *which combined unflagging comic invention with a scrupulous recreation of the American Civil War.*

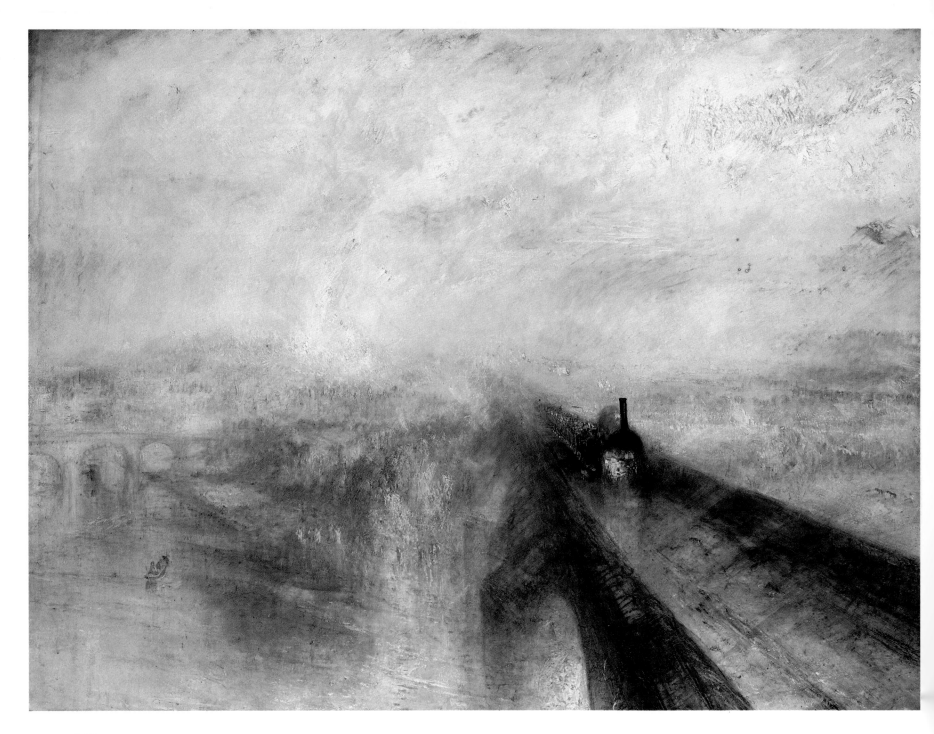

Opposite *J. M. W. Turner's vision of Brunel's bridge across the Thames at Maidenhead. 'Rain, Steam and Speed', painted as early as 1843, remains the definitive impression of rail travel.*

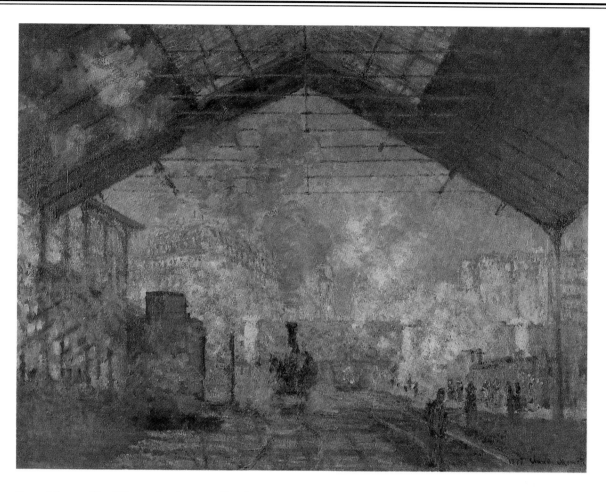

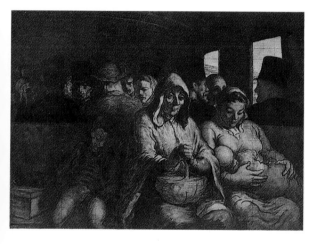

Honoré Daumier's realistic view of Third Class travel.

One of the results of the productive year Claude Monet spent painting at Saint Lazare station in Paris.

*T*he first art-form which took full advantage of the railways was the novel. Everything connected with the railways was inherently dramatic, the stations themselves provided admirable opportunities for selling the resulting books, and the journeys were equally suited to reading. Within two decades Fanny Kemble's sense of wonderment at the mere fact of travelling by rail had been transformed into a worldly weariness, a boredom which could most easily be relieved by the provision of solid reading matter during journeys which, in many cases, lasted days on end.

A handful of entrepreneurs, notably W. H. Smith in Britain and Louis Hachette in France, exploited the new appetites by opening bookstalls on the platforms of every major railway station. These supplied not only newspapers, but also magazines, many of them including novels in weekly or fortnightly parts. As a result the 'railway novel' was born. Novelists as distinguished as Charles Dickens obliged by supplying many of their novels in magazine-sized chunks – and publishers such as Routledge came up with series of books suitable for rail travellers.

The first generation of Victorian novelists were not great users of railway-related raw material, although railways, trains and journeys were woven into the stuff of life and thus appeared in the background of many of them. Of course, too, railway stations were ideal locations for dramatic suicides – like those of Tolstoy's Anna Karenina and of the adventurer Lopez in Trollope's *The Prime Minister*. Trollope sets the suicide at 'Tenway Junction', clearly modelled on Willesden Junction in north-west London, which until quite recently was just as dank and fearsome as it was in the novel a hundred years ago. Dickens also used a railway as the scene of a suicide, of the evil Carker in *Dombey and Son*. This novel, written during the great railway mania of 1845–6, is the only one of the age to take railways as a theme, almost a character in the story, for Dickens keeps returning to railways and railway journeys as symbols of death and destruction, of landscapes as of people.

A later generation of novelists exploited the aura of crime, sex and violence surrounding the new breed of luxury trains which emerged in the last decade of the nineteenth century. As we saw in Chapter 7 the association was epitomized by the Orient Express, with the innumerable films and novels about the crimes and passions

consummated on it, including a long-forgotten best-seller of the 1920s, Maurice Deko-
bra's *The Madonna of the Sleeping Car.*

Visually, later artists were unlucky that the first portrayal of a locomotive in motion, Turner's *Rail, Steam and Speed*, was one of the greatest paintings of all time, an extraordinary precursor of Impressionism. Remarkably, considering the nature of the painting, it was based on a real incident. The image was created when a sudden squall erupted on a journey from Exeter to London. A certain Lady Simon, who happened to be in the same compartment as Turner, described him as:

> ... an elderly gentleman, short and stout, with a red face and a curious prominent nose. [He was] ... strangely excited when a violent storm swept over the country, blotting out the sunshine and the blue sky and hanging like a pall over the landscape ... a train was coming in their direction, through the blackness, over one of Brunel's bridges, and the effect of the locomotive, lit by the crimson flame and seen through driving rain and whirling tempest, gave a peculiar impression of power, speed and stress.

Turner's extraordinary image naturally encouraged later artists: Camille Pissarro, for example, contributed some fine paintings of railways in South London during his exile there following the Franco-Prussian War. As Louis Armand, greatest of twentieth-century railwaymen, pointed out, every school of artists found inspiration in railways:

> The Impressionists fixed on forms moving through the countryside and on the wisps of steam which provide movement in even the most tranquil sky. The Fauves discovered an imposing force in the railways which provided the effect of weightiness they were looking for. More modern artists have perceived in the railways an ensemble of lines and curves which responded to the new rules of painting. All of them have found something to take because the train, the station, the tracks themselves are all parts of living reality.

But the greatest railway paintings inevitably transcend reality. It was natural for the Impressionists to concentrate on the Gare St Lazare and the line leading to Rouen and Normandy. They habitually met at a little café above the approaches to the station, and took their holidays on the Normandy coast. Monet's great series on the station used it and the locomotives as pretexts for celebrations of their romantic power and not (as Ruskin would probably have wished) as symbols of industrial brutality.

Because railways were so intimately linked with every aspect of people's lives they inspired satirists and cartoonists as surely and as permanently as 'fine' artists. As a result cartoons drawn of 'railway situations' provide an incomparable picture of people's relationship with them – and, especially, the initial hostility inspired by their owners, directors, and, above all, promoters. The hostility naturally came to a head with the attacks on the so-called Railway King, George Hudson, and the other shady luminaries of the Great Railway Mania of 1845–6. One artist did a splendid series on 'How he reigned and how he mizzled'. John Tenniel, now remembered mainly for his illustrations to the works of Lewis Carroll, attacked the railways since he felt it was his 'mission to strike at fraud and corruption' which he saw epitomized by the railways and their bosses.

For a century or more *Punch*, that reliable barometer of British middle-class taste, was full of railway cartoons. When the magazine was young and radical, these were often vicious attacks on the railways' bosses, like those drawn by Tenniel. But then they mellowed into cosier images. These often involved the supposed quaintness of the behaviour of railway porters and guards – the workers were a never-ending cause for condescending mirth (I remember how, as recently as 1961, Alan Bennett made the words 'a servant of the railway company' sound irresistibly droll). Other reliable standbys were the problems associated with losing your luggage, or being confined with a tiresome 'character' in a railway compartment during a long journey.

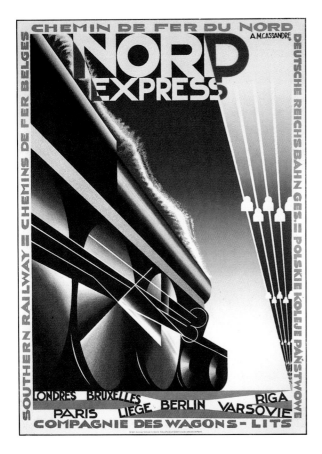

The French artist A. M. Cassandre perfectly encapsulated the glamour of international rail travel between the wars.

*T*he railways themselves naturally produced their own publicity material, often in the form of guides to the routes they traversed. The British companies were early in the field – as early as 1887 the Cambrian railway tried to entice travellers on to their normally unprofitable lines through mid-Wales with the publication of the provocatively-titled *What to See and Where to Stay in Wild Wales*. In 1907 the London & North Western went further by commissioning a film on North Wales, romantically entitled *The Land of Castles and Waterfalls*.

It was the American companies, with really wild scenery to offer, which could

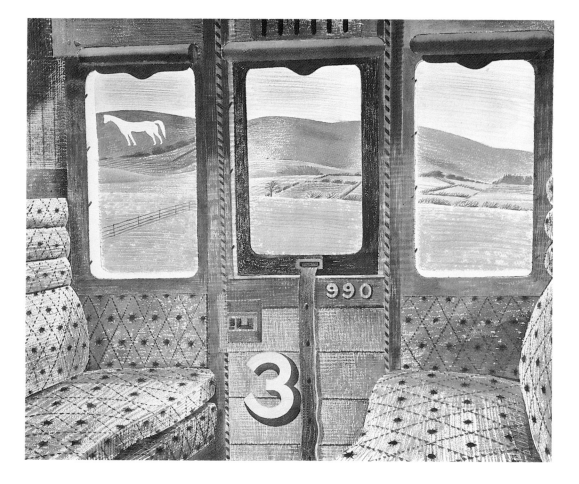

Eric Ravilous captured the Englishman's ideal view from a railway carriage – a white horse on the Wiltshire Downs.

legitimately go the furthest: indeed the record, for solidity anyway, was probably held by the New York Central's guide, *Health and Pleasure on America's Greatest Railroad*, its 552 pages weighing in at almost 1 kg (2 lb).

The railways were also lavish publishers of posters (which they could display on their own premises without any outlay) and were naturally early exploiters of another technical invention of the mid-nineteenth century, photography, to record and publicize their activities and the destinations they served. In the twentieth century many of the most vivid images provided by the advertising business came from the major railway companies, notably in France, where the images produced by artists like Cassandre immortalized the expresses used by British travellers going to Paris and onwards to the Riviera.

*I*n the United States the locomotives, the trains, the tracks, indeed everything to do with the railway, became the raw material for every type of folk art. According to Seymour Dunbar (in *A History of Travel in America, Vol. I*):

> Crude representations of railroad locomotives and cars began to appear as decorative patterns on the dishes, china and glassware used by the people. Small metallic medals were struck in honor of the introduction of the railroad. The popular sheet-music of the period was occasionally embellished with pictures of steam-engines and cars. Even whisky bottles appeared bearing upon their sides crude designs and inscriptions commemorating the introduction of railed tracks.

Artists, architects and the railways blended to the greatest effect in two major urban metropolitan systems. Best known is the contribution made by Frank Pick, not only to the London Transport system, but to the philosophy of the importance of art and design in metropolitan transport systems in general.

Pick was a man of an extraordinary breadth of vision. He joined the Underground group in 1906 and two years later was given the job of improving its then poor public image. One of his first steps was to inaugurate a poster campaign to publicize the Underground's service and to encourage travel, and throughout the next thirty years he deliberately employed the best artists of the period for the purpose. But he went much further, ensuring that the stations contained special display areas so that the posters were visible to travellers, and he employed Eric Gill, a typographical genius, to adapt the clear, legible, elegant typeface still in use today from an original design by Edward Johnston. He exploited the extensions of the Underground built in the 1930s to widen the range of passengers and their destinations, notably by luring them far out into the countryside round London. A great believer in the integrated approach to design, he introduced a standard type of station which combined the elegance of the Modern movement with the homeliness, the practicality of older English architectural traditions, resulting in a series of sturdy, practical but elegant buildings.

Unfortunately less appreciated, except by the travellers still using them, are the splendid architectural achievements of Hector Guimard, one of the prophets of Art

Nouveau, epitomized by the many stations he designed for the Paris Métro. Because the system was built all of a piece, Paris is still studded with hundreds of stations, all recognizable from their splendidly ornamented cast-iron entrances, which he called his edicules. His work was so innovatory – and so all-pervasive – that for a time Art Nouveau was actually known as *le style Métro*.

In Britain the four major rail companies formed in 1923 also advanced the use of art in railway publicity. The Southern used every visual device in what the *Railway Gazette* called 'a systematic scheme of connected and co-related publicity.' The London & North Eastern Railway used Eric Gill to design a special typeface, and put a number of leading artists under contract to produce posters. The biggest system, the London, Midland and Scottish, went even further, asking eighteen Royal Academicians to produce designs for posters. All (except Frank Brangwyn, who was already working for the LNER) accepted, and only Augustus John failed to come up with a design. While other major companies (notably Shell) adopted the same policy, the size of the railway companies – and the opportunity they offered to display artists' work – made them the leading sponsors of fine commercial art between the wars.

Unfortunately nationalization, the systematic starving of finance and sheer lack of imagination has meant that the tradition has largely died out. Moreover the battle for the soul of railway art, waged between modernists and realists in the 1920s and 1930s to the great benefit of the travelling public, was decisively won by the realists after the war. Indeed the most popular 'railway artist' in post-war Britain is Terence Cuneo, painter of hundreds of detailed but glamorized, romantically-enhanced visions of steam trains, a perfect emblem of the backward-looking attitude of British rail-lovers in the past forty years.

Railways, and indeed everything to do with them, were inherently theatrical but theatres were not ideal venues for dramatizing railway themes. Yet, as early as 1844, an enterprising manager put on the first 'railway play' in which the heroine – peering through a convenient grating – sees a man lying across the rails. Such plays were followed by slide shows which portrayed railways the world over.

These were sometimes extremely elaborate. One of the hits of the 1900 Universal Exhibition in Paris was a panorama devised by a Polish artist called Piatsetski. Spectators would sit in a make-believe railway carriage, and through the windows they would see a long series of images (still preserved in the Hermitage Museum in St Petersburg) representing a train journey from that city to Peking. The end of the performance was signalled by a guard announcing that the train had arrived at Peking.

The idea was probably based on a display devised by George C. Hale, a former chief of the Kansas City Fire Brigade, itself inspired by the popularity of films showing a fire brigade turning out. At the 'tour' he exhibited in Oxford Street in London you could go on a 'trip through the Rocky Mountains', complete with a 'conductor' taking the fares, and suitable noises like the hiss of escaping steam. When stations were passed the car (mounted on an elaborate suspension system to imitate the ride on a train) would slow up, and bells would sound. Within a few years Hale made £2 million, a gigantic sum at the time.

The true glory of the train as an inherent part of a major art-form had to await the coming of the cinema. The cinema was made for trains. Indeed some observers have seen the two experiences, of travel by train and watching a film, as very similar. Both are unnatural, both are alienating, cutting you off from your environment and removing any control over it. Both involve the initially disconcerting experience of watching a rapidly changing series of images which, however, can add up to a total experience. With a film, of course, the sequence is deliberately designed to tell a story but even the apparently 'accidental' sequence involved in a railway journey involves a gradual transition through a world, a civilization, a landscape, designed by nature or by man.

Even better for the film-makers are the natural excitement of a locomotive, the equally obvious fact that a station was the proper location for dramatic or emotional arrivals and farewells, and that journeys often involved groups of strangers being cooped up together for days on end. In the last ninety years the visual imagination and artistic and philosophical creativity of film-makers world-wide have exploited the possibilities in so many ways that they are difficult to categorize.

The film industry first used trains and stations because they were by far the most dramatic element in the daily lives of potential customers, though a familiar one. The first films were simply designed to show the power of moving, as opposed to static, images, so not surprisingly trains were seen as a perfect vehicle.

In the late 1890s the first demonstration of 'moving images' was Louis Lumière's *Train Leaving a Station*. Then in 1902 the Lackawanna and Delaware Western railroad staked an important place in the history of the cinema when it commissioned a film from Edwin S. Porter, a young technician working for the Edison company. The film, entitled *The Romance of the Rails*, plugged the virtues of the self-styled Road of Anthracite, for the railroad used a fuel which was not only mined along the route, but had the undeniable advantage that it was relatively smokeless. Some anonymous publicity genius dreamed up a fictional character called Phoebe Snow who sang:

> *I won my fame and wide acclaim*
> *For Lackawanna's splendid name*
> *By keeping bright and snowy white*
> *Upon the Road of Anthracite.*

The following year, inspired by the success of an advertisement which remained embedded in the American subconscious for generations, Porter went on to make a film which became the very first box-office hit, *The Great Train Robbery*.

Ever since, trains, tracks and stations have been the natural scene of films of all kinds. The early days of Hollywood saw innumerable series, all very similar. *The Perils of Pauline*, with Pearl White eternally tied to the tracks as the express thunders towards her lovely and helpless body, soon found imitators with names like *The Hazards of Helen* – all filmed on the nearby Santa Fe tracks.

As early as 1914 Vitagraph staged the first real-life filmed crash for the appropriately-named film, *The Wreck*, at a cost of £10,000. But then virtually every name in the early history of the cinema seems either to have made a specifically railway film or to have used tracks, stations or trains as locations. In 1911 D. W. Griffith directed *The Lonedale Operator – A dramatic account of a railway crash averted at the last moment* and even after his fall from grace the great comedian Fatty Arbuckle directed a comedy called *The Iron Mule*.

For half a century afterwards film-makers all over the world made full use of train locations, either to create a suitably dramatic atmosphere, often in a film's opening sequence, or as the scene for an exciting final sequence. The list is endless: from the menacing arrival of the stranger, perhaps most powerfully evoked in *Bad Day at Black Rock* or *3.10 to Yuma*, to the unseen power of the railroad barons – the only posse which strikes fear into the hearts of Butch Cassidy and the Sundance Kid is the one financed by a man they describe simply as 'Mr Harriman'.

Britain's two most successful film directors were both fully aware of the usefulness of trains and stations. David Lean exploited T. E. Lawrence's demolition job on the Hejaz railway to the full, but perhaps the most exciting single railway-related sequence in any British film is the end of Carol Reed's film about an IRA informer, *Odd Man Out*.

It is set in a marshalling yard. These were ideal locations for chases, especially in the days when films were mostly shot in black and white. Because the lighting was fierce but high and distant, the contrast between light and shadow was naturally (but by normal standards unnaturally) sharp; this, combined with the noises, above all the metallic clanking of the wagons as they banged together, made the yard the natural venue for the chase at the end of the film. A similarly exciting chase comes at the end of *49th Parallel*, a classic spy thriller starring Leslie Howard.

Chases were, usually, merely individual sequences. Films which revolved entirely around a railway setting were another matter. In his invaluable book *The Railways on the Screen* John Huntley makes a key distinction: 'In Europe railway films of the 1930s tended to be of the "people thrown together on a train" type whereas the Americans relied largely on, more or less dramatized, true stories.' He could usefully have added that each culture reflected the train in its own way.

Perhaps the three most typically British railway films could not have been conceived in any other cultural environment. David Lean's *Brief Encounter* famously makes use of the station as the stage for chance meeting, the drabness of the wartime setting combining agonizingly with the limitless English capacity for understatement, the native inability

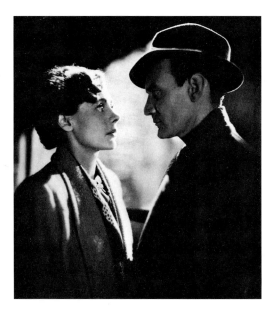

If you have tears prepare to shed them now: Celia Johnson and Trevor Howard in David Lean's 1946 film Brief Encounter.

to express strong emotions except in the most stilted of forms. He used another English failing, the overly-conscientious sense of duty exploited for inherently evil purposes, in *Bridge Over the River Kwai*. At a lower level, Will Hays' film *Oh Mr Porter* is a deeply satisfying exploration of all the jokes possible about the generally unamusing 'characters' who worked for railways. And if it's national attitudes you want, the backward-looking British attitude to railways since the Second World War is perfectly epitomized by the most insufferably twee of all the films made by Ealing Studios, *The Titfield Thunderbolt*, a whimsical account of the attempted rescue of a rural railway line.

These lines had symbolized the tranquillity of the Edwardian rural dream ever since it was shattered by the horrors of the First World War, so they naturally bred poems as well as films. Perhaps the purest example is *There's Peacetime in That Train* by Edward

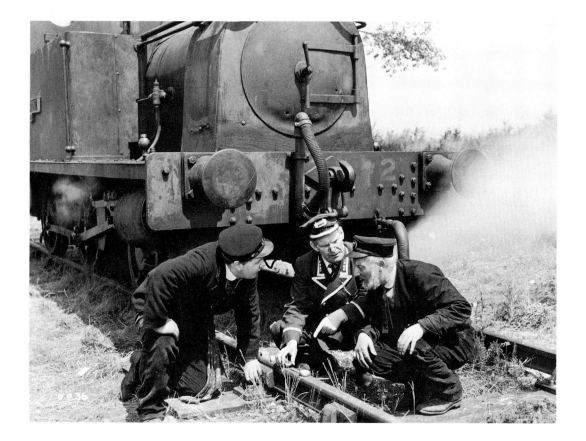

The greatly underrated Will Hay, with his accomplices Moore Marriott and Graham Moffatt in his 1938 masterpiece Oh! Mr Porter.

Thomas, in which the poet finds solace in the familiar noise of a train rumbling past the fields. But the best-known is another of Thomas's poems *Adlestrop* which, in reality as well as poesy, is indeed a magically peaceful station, set in the middle of nowhere. (I can vouch for the essential truthfulness of his poem, since a steam train in which I was travelling *did* stop for no apparent reason at Adlestrop one sunny Sunday afternoon in June, some forty years ago.)

The Americans were always aware of the role railroads had played in their history. Perhaps the most typical (if not the most distinguished) cinematic result was Cecil B. de Mille's film *Union Pacific*, portraying the construction of the first American trans-continental railroad. But it was individual characters, individual incidents, which provided the opportunity for most American 'railroad movies.' These ranged from a real-life railroad robbery in *Denver and Rio Grande* to *The Harvey Girls* of 1936. This, a famous movie in its time, was the true story of how Fred Harvey brought good food to every stop the length of the Atchison Topeka and Santa Fe, with the help of the Harvey Girls, respectable young ladies who waited at table and soon found husbands. The movie was chiefly notable for one of the 'Girls', played by Judy Garland, singing that eternal show-stopper, 'The Atchison Topeka and the Santa Fe'.

An exception to all the rules, simply a film which combines all the elements connected with railways and the people who work on them, is Jean Renoir's film version of Emile Zola's novel, *La Bête Humaine*. It tells the story of Jacques Lantier, a young engine driver (played by Jean Gabin) who is subject to murderous brainstorms. It culminates in an almost unbearably exciting final sequence in which Lantier, on the footplate of the Paris express, confesses to his fireman, overpowers him, and finally plunges to his death off the tender, leaving the train to race on to its doom. This film really has everything, including the luscious Simone Simon as the wife of a jealous stationmaster who murders her elderly lover in an almost empty train.

But Huntley is right in suggesting that European directors preferred to exploit the inherent drama and claustrophobia when a group of dissimilar people are on a train together. As early as 1933 Anatole Litvak's *Sleeping Car* portrays an improbable romance set on an express thundering across Europe.

Opposite *Jean Gabin as the murderous engine driver, Jacques Lantier, in Jean Renoir's 1938 film version of Emile Zola's classic novel* La Bête Humaine.

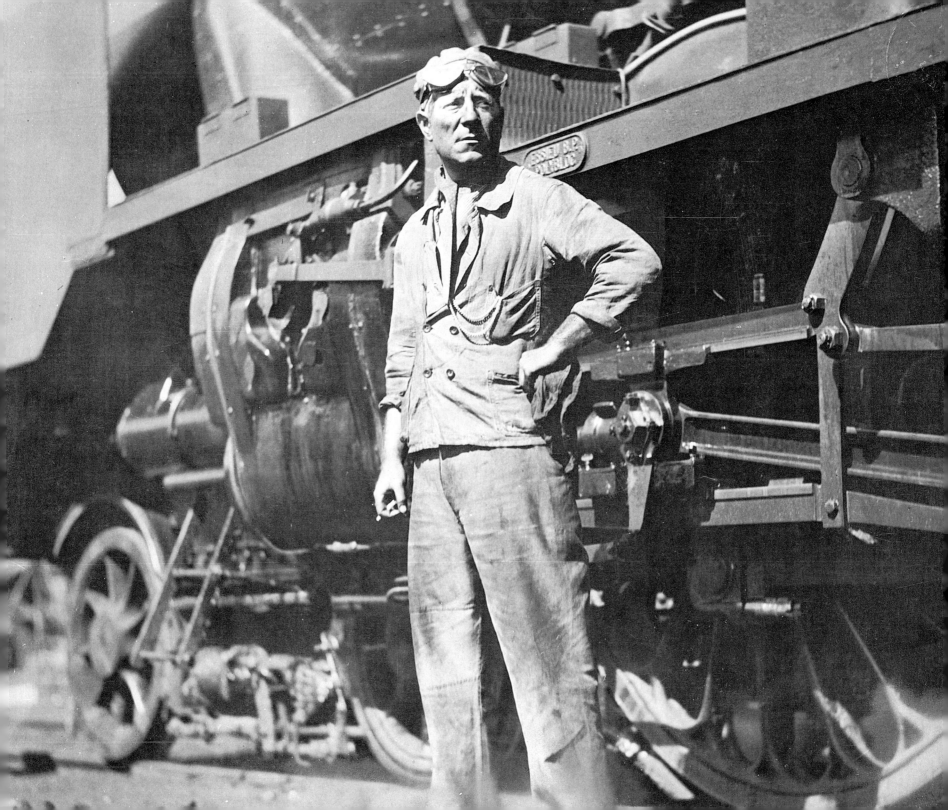

Eroticism incarnate in Hitchcock's 1959 film
North By North West: *Cary Grant and Eve Marie Saint line up for the longest kiss in screen history, which ends only when the train enters a tunnel.*

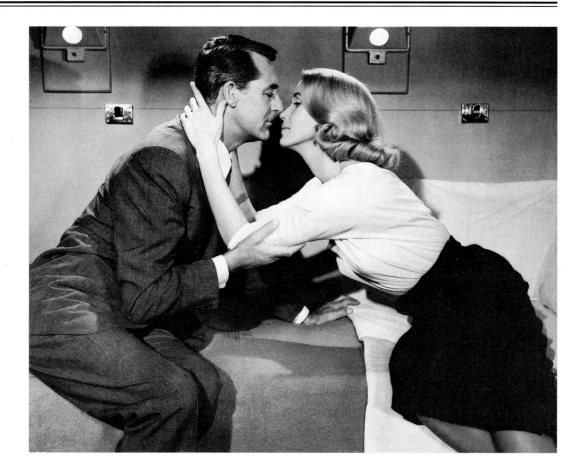

But for me – and all such choices must in the end be personal, must depend on one's judgement, not only of the worth of the film, but of the importance of the 'railway element' – all the conditions for 'railway greatness' are most amply fulfilled by two very different films, which could be said to sum up the American and European traditions respectively, Buster Keaton's *The General* and Alfred Hitchcock's *The Lady Vanishes*.

In *The General* the locomotive of the title is one of the most important characters, without in any way becoming mawkish. It is there, it matters – to the hero, the Confederate engineer Johnny Gray – as well as to the film. The story is closely based on a real incident during the Civil War when a group of Unionist soldiers infiltrated the Confederate lines and nearly managed to cut the army's main line of communication. But they were foiled by a Confederate engineer and fireman who successfully chased the train the Unionist soldiers had commandeered.

Keaton's hero is anxious to demonstrate to his loved one that he is worthy of her after she had spurned him as a coward because he had not been allowed to fight. And the depth of the feeling he can show without moving a muscle is matched by his extraordinary ingenuity in exploiting the comic possibilities inherent in the chase. Its reality greatly heightened the effectiveness of the movie. By contrast the mayhem when the Brothers wreck a train in the *The Marx Brothers Go West* looks strained and artificial. Keaton is also far more successful in recreating the atmosphere of the South during the War than was David O. Selznick in *Gone with the Wind*. But then, as Keaton is alleged to have said: 'They went to a novel for their story, I went to history.'

In another personal choice, I find that it is Alfred Hitchcock who provides the perfect people-on-a train movie in *The Lady Vanishes*. Hitchcock was always fond of trains, using them again for sinister purposes in *Strangers on a Train*, and to convey sex in *North-by-Northwest* where the hero and heroine get together on a train which then passes through a long, simplistically Freudian tunnel.

The Lady Vanishes is adapted from a novel (*The Wheel Spins*, by Ethel Lina White) and set on a train travelling through central Europe. It is a prolonged metaphor for British attitudes towards the looming menace of Hitler, ranging from the acceptance of the threat by the heroine, a doughty old lady played by Dame May Whitty, to the insouciance of the comics Basil Radford and Naunton Wayne. The film is that rarest of works, a comedy-thriller backed by an iron moral fist in the funniest and most thrilling of gloves. All that and splendid steam locomotives too.

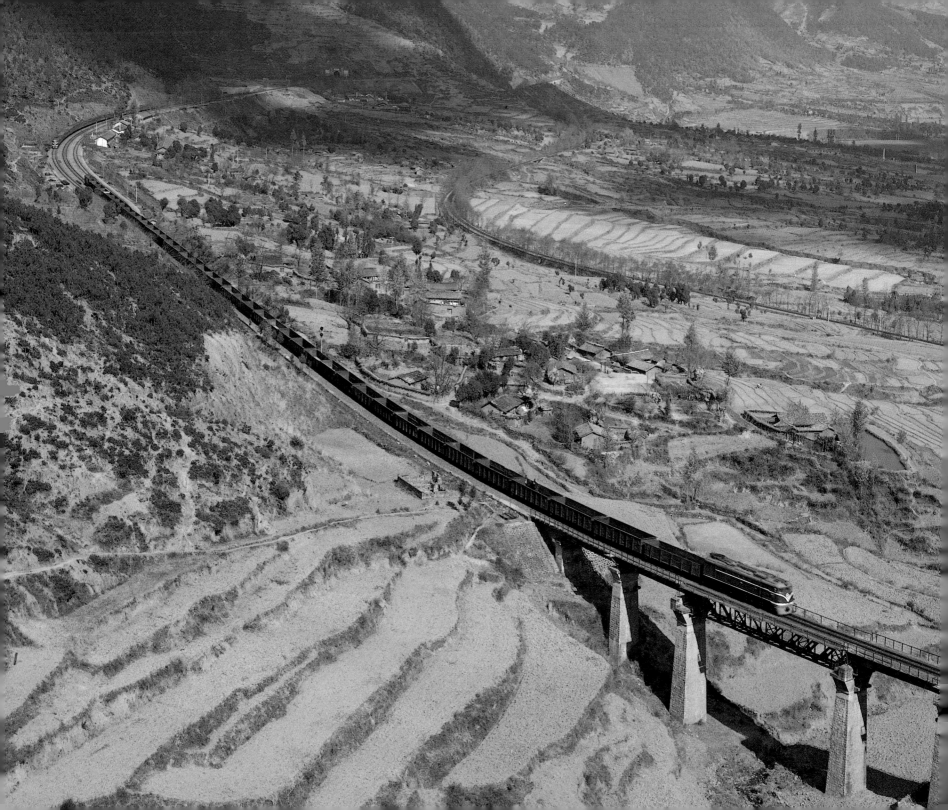

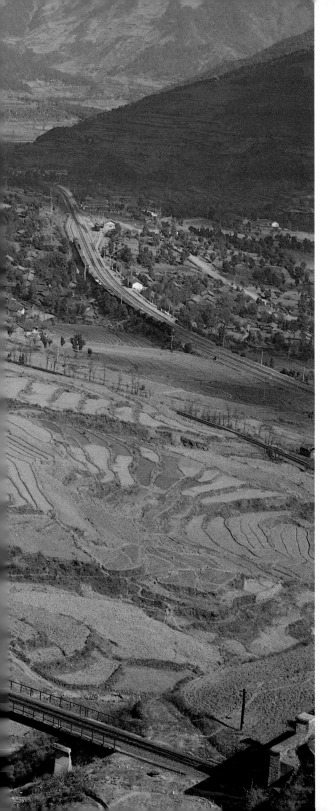

10   *Return Train*

F or nearly three decades after 1945 railways seemed doomed to play an ever-decreasing role in people's lives. Even Arthur C. Clarke, whose prophecies proved uncannily right so often, got it wrong. Although he envisaged trains as playing a major role in freight transport, he prophesied in 1964 (in *Profile of the Future*) that passengers would use other means of transport.

Throughout the world institutional rigidities prevented railways from adapting to challenge the increasing domination of the car, the lorry and the bus. Yet in the past thirty years the railways have started to fight back. The age of the all-conquering motor car and truck is over and, as forecast forty years ago by the late Louis Armand, the train looks likely to be the key means of land transport for the twenty-first century as it was for the nineteenth.

Moreover, and this is even more surprising, the new trains are still powered by electric motors (or even, in the case of heavy long-distance freight, diesels) and are carried on steel wheels running on steel rails. The old combination has proved far more adaptable than anyone dreamed possible a generation ago, and since then many once-promising alternatives have fallen by the wayside.

The use of gas turbines or jet engines, which seemed a promising development in the 1960s, was abruptly halted by the oil crisis of 1973, which brought the cost of fuel far more to the forefront of the transport equation, and thus militated in favour of electricity as motive power. Early attempts to use hovercraft operating on a cushion of air foundered

On the rugged line between Kunming and Chengdu, one of the many built by the Chinese since 1949.

203

at the same time. The only competitor now in the field involves the use of magnetic force to keep the train above the ground, thus permitting speeds of up to 650 kph (400 mph). Unfortunately no one has yet solved the most difficult problem, that of ensuring that the track above which the train rises is laid with the required precision over long distances. And even if this problem is solved, magnetic levitation – or Maglev as it is generally known – is fighting a rapidly-moving competitive target.

When the Tokaido line in Japan, the first 'super-train', started running in October 1964, the trains averaged a mere 160 kph (100 mph). Today the French are operating trains as a matter of course at average speeds of over 240 kph (160 mph), and there seems no reason why an average of 320 kph (200 mph) will not be commonplace on new lines before the end of the century.

This acceptance of the inherent perfectibility of well-proved techniques fits in with other trends, notably the acceptance of the internal combustion engine as the motive power for land-based vehicles, and for such 'old-fashioned' aircraft as the jumbo jet as the standard means of inter-continental transport.

*I*n a few countries the government never lost faith in the railway, largely because the basic network was still not complete. The most obvious case was China, where, as we saw in Chapter 5, the idea of 'self-built' railways had been an article of revolutionary faith for over half a century before the Communists took over in 1949. In the course of the next twenty-five years the new government completed the network, covering even the western half of the country with new lines.

The insistence on railways as a primary means of revolutionary development was not surprising. Sun Yat-Sen, the leader of the 1911 Revolution, had always been obsessed by railways. When he was pushed aside after the Revolution he was quite happy to be given the purely nominal job of planning a new railway network for his country. His ideas seemed fanciful at the time, but provided a model for his successors.

To the Chinese their own railways were firm proof that they had indeed escaped from colonial control. In the 1930s and 1940s this had been largely Japanese control. They had treated the railways in Manchuria as a 'Great Civilizing Agent' after their conquest in the 1930s (and true to their word, provided some of the fastest train services in the world). Although the Japanese left the lines in the territory they occupied in good shape, the civil war between 1945 and 1949 left the Communist victors with a derelict system which reached only the eastern half of their country.

Mao Tse-Tung was as interested as Sun Yat-Sen in railways, but his priorities were political, not economic. Far from concentrating on improving the lines between developed centres he pushed the railways west and north into China's far-flung Far West in a successful attempt to control all these provinces. He remembered how warlords had escaped central control largely because of the lack of communications, and how he had been able to escape from a revengeful central government through his Long March into the wilderness. The result was, ironically a classic 'Imperial' railway system, providing a means of central control far more complete than that achieved by the 'capitalist imperialist' powers.

The construction rate was startling, matching or improving on the great days of earlier transcontinental systems. In barely more than a decade after the Communist triumph in 1949 the Chinese built over 12,000 miles (19,000 km) of new railways while repairing another 4000.

Like their nineteenth century predecessors, the Chinese relied almost entirely on human muscle power. According to a CIA estimate, up to 1.3 million Chinese were working on railway construction in the mid-1950s, only one in seven a permanent railway employee. The remainder were press-ganged into work brigades. And, like their predecessors, they died in their thousands. In *Riding the Red Rooster* Paul Theroux wrote how one cemetery contained:

> ... the graves of the men who died while building the railway, it took ten years. These ten years from the early 1960s to the 1970s coincided with the period of patriotic fervour and intense jingoism. It not only had the largest number of self-sacrificing soldiers and workers, but also an enormous number of political prisoners. The efforts of those passionate people produced this Chengdu-Kunming line.

It was an extraordinary achievement. Its 600 miles (965 km) required 440 tunnels (some of them spirals to cope with the gradients) and 653 bridges, covering a total of

Return Train

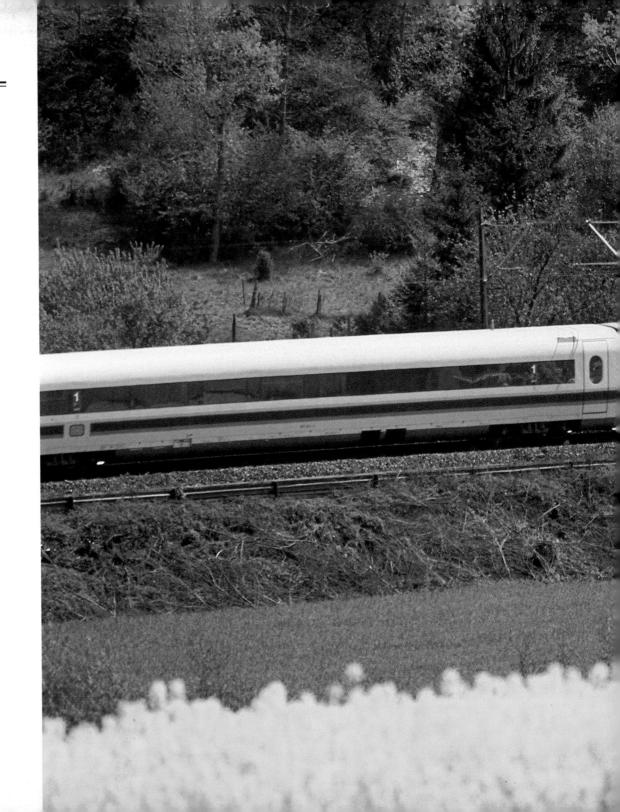

The ICE, Germany's ultra-fast answer to the French TGV, rushing through the peaceful countryside of Baden-Würtemburg.

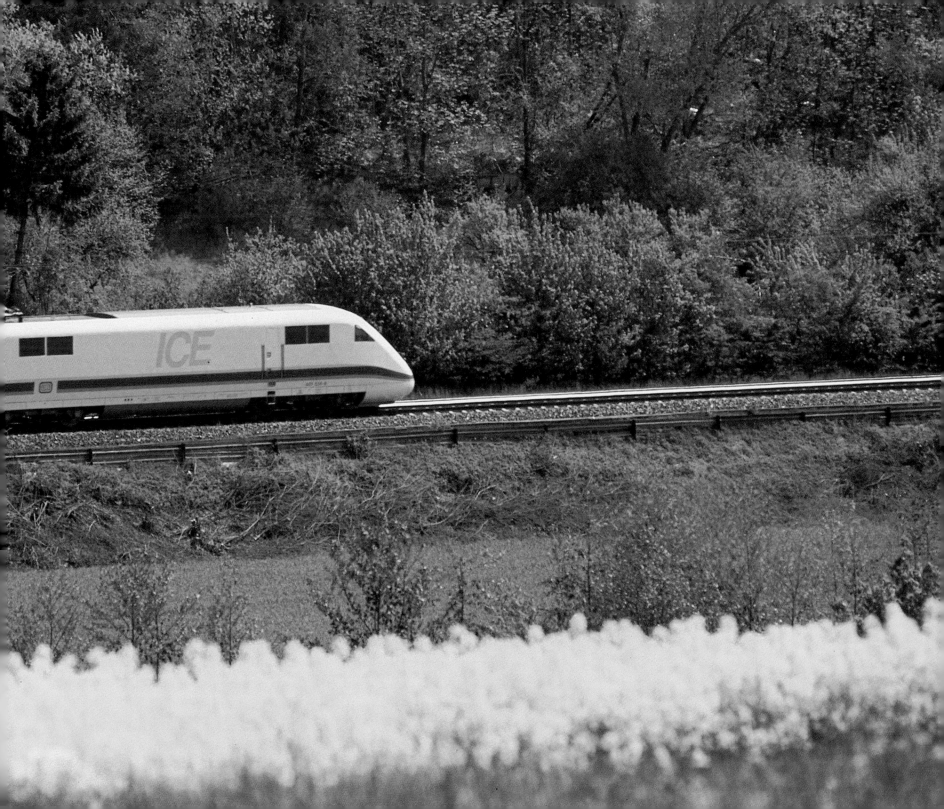

278 miles (477 km) of forests and mountains, gorges and swift-flowing rivers. Even more remarkable was the 569 mile (916 km) line north from the old nationalist capital of Chongqing to Xiangfan, a line with 716 bridges and 400 tunnels. But the culminating achievement of these Chinese Imperial railways came with the 1400–mile (2253–km) route to Golmud in Tibet on the road to Lhasa where, according to Patrick and Maggy Whitehouse in *China by Rail* the trains 'carry a doctor with oxygen apparatus to assist those whose respiratory systems fail to cope with the rareified atmosphere.' Equally extraordinary were the great bridges over the Yangtse at Wuhan and at Nanjing, one of the wonders of the world. The Whitehouses describe how:

> Trains travel inside its vaulted metal girders for a journey of four miles across the river itself and another three on the approaches from either side ... the sensation is similar to becoming airborne, looking down at first on narrow fields, on ponds and tracks, with tiny people tilling and harvesting, and then crossing the broad, grey waters of the inland sea, dotted with cargo ships and fishing boats bobbing and heaving in the wake of the industrial traffic.

After the pioneering period (and the Cultural Revolution which merely slowed railway construction) came an equally intensive phase of modernization, replacing steam engines with diesels, electrifying major lines, double-tracking others. The investment remained enormous, if only because traffic had grown at such a rate. By 1975 freight traffic was sixteen times the 1949 level and has increased just as rapidly since then. But as China's economy grows by leaps and bounds so the rail system is stretched to breaking point especially in the south east, where capacity will need to double in the 1990s to meet even pessimistic forecasts of the demand.

Much of the developing world, most obviously the newly-independent countries of southern Africa, shared the Chinese vision of railways as the prime symbol of industrial progress. This was vividly and appropriately demonstrated by the so-called Tazara railway. This was a perfect example of the failure of colonialism to retain its power against the newly-independent African states, able to use the modern equivalent of the Great Game, the world-wide battle for influence between the capitalist west and the Communists.

In the mid-1950s President Nasser of Egypt had overcome the American refusal to finance the Aswan Dam by calling in the Russians. Ten years later it was the turn of the Chinese to come to the help of the Zambians and the Tanzanians after the World Bank had refused to finance the Tazara, a new rail line from the port of Dar-es-Salaam in Tanzania through to the copper belt in Zambia.

In the early 1960s the price of copper rose to an all-time high, and the problems of transporting the metal from Zambia, at the time the third largest producer in the world, became immense, espcially after Ian Smith, then Prime Minister of Southern Rhodesia, had declared UDI in 1965. 'Tiny' Rowland, the Chairman of the trading group, Lonrho, came up with the idea of a new railway to the Indian Ocean, drawing a straight line on the map to show Kenneth Kaunda, then Prime Minister of Zambia, the way. According to Kaunda, the imperial powers: 'wanted us to continue to be dependant on the existing railway . . . through to South Africa.'

But Britain and the World Bank remained opposed to the scheme throughout. And

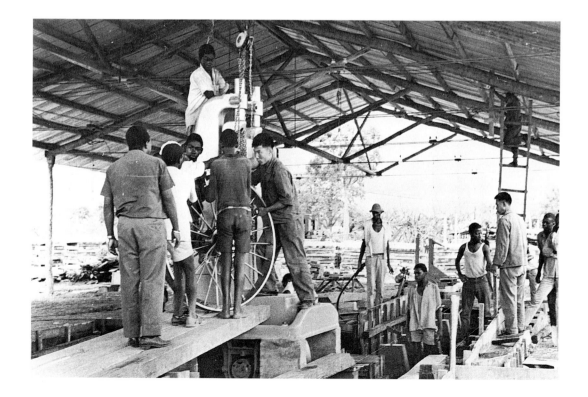

Another Chinese triumph: building the Tanzam railway from Dar-Es-Salaam to the Zambian copper mines.

the Bank never gave further work to a British consultancy, Maxwell Stamp Associates, which had reported in its favour.

Despite vague gestures of support from some western governments, the decision to accept help from the Chinese was made after a visit to Peking by President Kaunda of Zambia in January 1967. Two years later the inhabitants of Dar-es-Salaam were astounded at the sight of a thousand Chinese in shapeless Mao suits with identical blue canvas suitcases marching in tightly-disciplined formation from their ship.

It cost the Chinese £169 million, and accounted for half their foreign aid budget. But it became a splendid propaganda weapon: 'It allowed them an entry into this part of the world with a massive show of planning and management of a big project' in the words of Andrew Kashita, the Zambian Minister of Transport. The first 480-km (300-mile) stretch was completed by November 1971 and the first trains ran over the entire route in November 1975, ahead of schedule.

Commemorating Mao Ze Dong, who built thousands of miles of railways to help him tighten his grip over China.

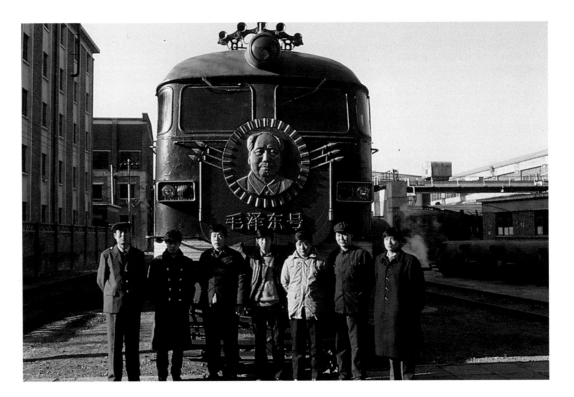

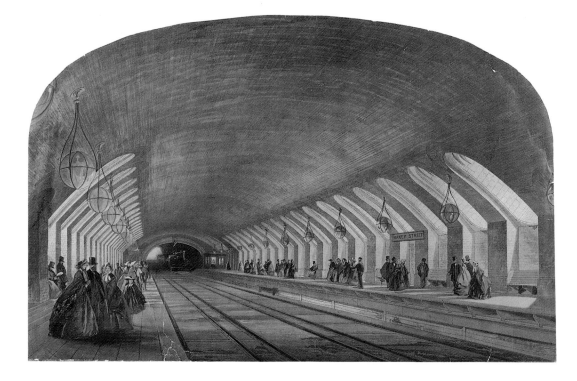

Baker Street Station on the first underground railway in the world, restored to its pristine splendour in the early 1980s. Note the air vents to let out the steam.

By contrast a road being built along the same route with American aid was six months late – and the surface broke up as a result of the first spring rains. Socially, too, the Chinese proved model ambassadors, behaving impeccably. Anxious not to be a burden they brought – or cultivated – their own food and lived by themselves. As a result of their discipline there were none of the babies of mixed blood which were an inevitable result of the influx of other races.

In the end even the sceptics had to cheer. As *The Times* put it: 'If Chinese influence has been gained, it has been earned.' For a time the Tazara proved immensely useful. In the late 1970s and most of the 1980s over four-fifths of Zambian exports ran over the railways. But soon the Tazara was plagued with problems: the engines broke down, there were constant landslides in southern Tanzania, and the port at Dar-es-Salaam remained chaotic. At the end of the 1980s the track was upgraded and new German locomotives have been bought, echoing the experience of earlier pioneering railways where the original line had to be strengthened within a couple of decades. But the end of apartheid, and the subsequent return of South Africa to its natural economic leadership in the region, has had an ironic effect, with the Zambians increasingly preferring to use the older-established (and far more efficient) rail links to South Africa.

*I*n countries with already developed networks the obstacles facing the railways were seemingly unsurmountable. They were faced by the sheer flexibility and apparent freedom of the internal combustion engine, and the very considerable state funding enjoyed by roads the world over. Then came the oil crisis of 1973–4 with its sudden transformation of the economics of transport in favour of relatively light users of fuel like the railways. But even more important was a change of mood. For it was only when the 'limits of growth' appeared, in the form of ever-increasing traffic jams and their accompanying pollution, that the train could really start to make an impact, that people and thus politicians were prepared to finance the investments required to bring railways back to the foreground of the world's transport vision. The trend back to railways is naturally gathering pace as the 'me-first-ism' of the 1980s is replaced by the 'caring' 1990s, with their concern for the environment as well as people.

But until recently it seemed that in most countries the railways' inflexible, over-manned, sclerotic, under-funded services, often government-owned, always state-regulated, could never hope to match the attractions of the car or lorry – even though railway fares were usually kept uneconomically low to placate the minority which still travelled by train. Enabling the railways to compete has meant a long struggle to restructure the organizational framework within which they operate.

Over the past decade the institutional rigidities have been relaxed. The lead was taken by British Rail, with its separation of business sectors and development of specialist marketing departments, and by the British and the Swedes with their separation of the track and the trains which ran on it.

If these organizational reforms had been matched by adequate investment, then Britain would have a decent rail sysem today. But, sadly, Britain is now the only exception to the rule that, after an interval of a hundred years, industrialized countries again perceive the health of their railway system as a reliable indicator of their position in the international league table and are backing their beliefs with hard cash.

There are many reasons for the British neglect. Behind it is the terrifying national nostalgia which afflicts railways worse almost than any other field of national endeavour – if only because the country has such a splendid railway past to be nostalgic about. This leads to the natural, but crippling, assumption that the country's great days, in terms of railways (as in so many aspects of British life), are irretrievably past.

The national lassitude was compounded by Mrs Thatcher, the arch-individualist, who despised railways as perfect examples of communal travel. Her successors, anxious to prove themselves worthy of the Thatcherite mantle, decided to privatize the system, even though The Lady herself and her most loyal supporters (including the late Lord Ridley, when he was Secretary of State for Transport) judged that the railways were best left as a publicly-owned service. Moreover, privatization provides the perfect excuse to postpone an urgently-needed investment programme for Britain's railway system.

But the British nostalgia did have one happy result, a concentration on enhancing the value of the rich architectural heritage left by the railways. Not only in Britain have stations become a symbol of urban renewal, of pride in a city's past, of the determination not to succumb to the all-devouring motor car. In New York the loss of Penn Station in the mid-1960s was mourned more than that of most other landmarks. In London the loss of the Euston Arch (in itself a dumpy and unremarkable monument) in 1963 was the signal for the forces of preservation to gird up their loins, although they had done nothing a few years earlier when a much nobler monument, the Great Hall at Euston, had been pulled down. In Paris, twenty years later, and only after a generation of hesitation, the Gare d'Orsay was transformed into a magnificent museum, whereas the Halles, an equally splendid relic of nineteenth-century elegance, had been pulled down in the 1970s.

The finest example of this real (and symbolic) renewal is in London, where British Rail's anonymous architects have restored Liverpool Street Station in all its glory. They were able to use appropriately rich colours to enhance the ironwork, secure in the knowledge that it would not be obscured by smoke and steam. The newly-restored masterpiece forms part of an excellently-designed scheme, the Broadgate office development. Broadgate also scores over its American equivalents in that it is not simply a hollow example of pious restoration of an old building whose original use is forgotten.

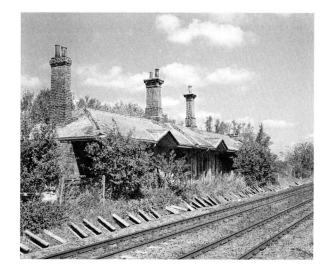

The end of the rural dream: the abandoned station at Brooksby in Leicestershire, built in 1846.

The British also took an early lead (which they have now, alas, lost) in the first and most obvious sign of the railways' renaissance, an almost universal improvement to existing lines. All over the world they are being restored and improved, services being speeded up, conditions improved. In the United States Amtrak, the skeletal national passenger service, has survived attacks during the Reagan years to emerge as an increasingly respected, if still minimal, contributor to the country's passenger transport services. Even the Japanese, the pioneers of new lines dedicated to passenger traffic, have also invested heavily in ordinary new trains and their infrastructure.

Moreover, systems in several countries are finding increasingly ingenious ways of improving speeds on unchanged infrastructure. The best example of such making-do is the tilting trains being introduced by the Spanish, the Italians and the Swedes to run far faster than before on existing lines – typically, an early British initiative with such trains was strangled by inadequate financing.

Far more glamorous are the handful of major new rail-related projects in developed countries providing long-dreamed-of links. Most obvious is the Chunnel, most ambitious the projected bridge-cum-tunnel connections between Denmark and Sweden and the new tunnels under the Alps due to open in the first decade of the twenty-first century. All, seemingly, are connected with the feeling that Europe needs the real unity to be found through tangible links like railways – a return, in fact, to the classic nineteenth-century philosophy – rather than through increasingly hollow declarations of forth-coming economic and political unity.

The most ambitious and expensive projects are the new tunnels under the Alps. These will pass under the very base of passes like the St Gotthard, rather than further up the slopes, like the present tunnels, which were dug in the second half of the nineteenth century. Obviously the lower the base point, the longer the tunnels, but the greater the savings in time and distance. The Swiss seem ready to finance the cost – in 1992 they voted enthusiastically in favour. The new route under the St Gotthard is worthy of the importance of this historic line, involving more than 160 km (100 miles) of new tracks and a tunnel over 48 km (30 miles) long.

Almost as large-scale are the bridges and tunnels designed to link Scandinavia with

Opposite Liverpool Street Station in London: perfectly restored by British Rail's anonymous and unsung architects in the late 1980s as part of the Broadgate office development.

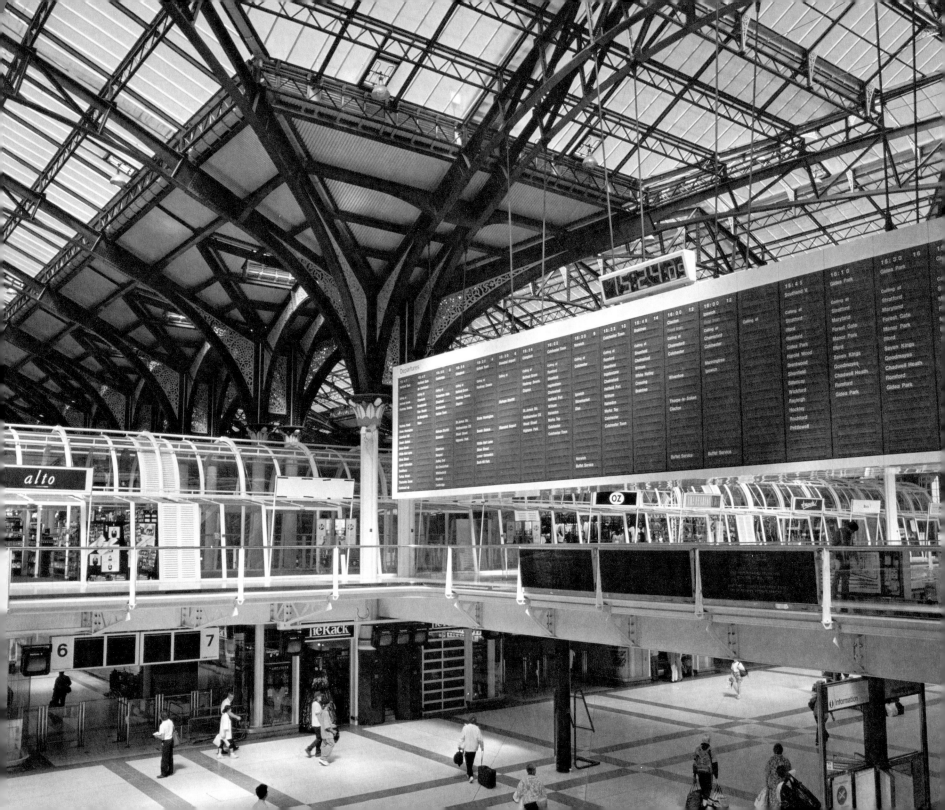

the European mainland, a series of schemes also fraught with socio-political significance. Just as the new Alpine tunnels symbolize the determination of the Swiss to remain the key land bridge between northern and southern Europe – while at the same time preserving their environment by forcing freight traffic off the roads onto the rails – so the new links across the Baltic demonstrate the determination of the Swedes and the Danes to forge increasing links with the rest of Europe and of the Germans to transform Berlin into the railway capital of Europe.

The first step in a triple project to link Scandinavia to the mainland of Europe crosses the Storebelt, the 'Great Belt' between the Danish mainland and Zealand – the island on which Copenhagen is built. The Danish Parliament twice blanched at the cost before passing the necessary legislation in 1987, possibly inspired by the progress on the Chunnel. It involves an 11 km (6.6 mile) bridge between the mainland and the small island of Sprogo, and a much longer bridge-plus-tunnel to span the 8 km (5 miles) between Sprogo and Zealand. The road bridge, with a main span of 6.8 km (4 miles), will be the longest suspension bridge in the world, and the rail tunnel (needed to prevent the bridge being unacceptedly heavy) second only to the Chunnel. Despite delays caused by labour disputes and by breakdowns to the tunnelling machines, the project should be completed by 1998.

The second stage consists of a bridge and tunnel link across the Oresund between Copenhagen and Malmö in Southern Sweden, due to be opened by the end of the century. The route was deliberately chosen in preference to a much shorter crossing 32 km (20 miles) to the north so as to create a new linear metropolis across the Oresund.

The new links will provide a – roundabout – rail link between Scandinavia and Germany, but the Germans are pressing for a speedy start on the third element in providing a direct route to the heart of Germany, a bridge-cum-tunnel from the Danish island of Lolland to the Fehmarn Peninsula in northern Germany. This would allow trains from Scandinavia to reach central Germany in under six hours, and at the same time boost Berlin's claim to be Europe's most important railway junction.

But most-publicized of all these projects is the tunnel under the English Channel. It was an absurdly long time a-building. First conceived in 1802 by one of Napoleon's engineers, it nearly became reality in the 1880s, when the last of the great megalomaniac British railway tycoons, Sir Edward Watkin, conceived of a Chunnel as a key link between the Continent and the north of England – indeed he built the Great Central line from Marylebone to Sheffield using the broader Continental loading gauge (although the rails remain 143.5 cm (4 ft 8½ in) apart the trains could be taller and broader). But his plans were quashed by the War Office, afraid of invasion by a lot of nasty foreigners.

This vague fear – expressed publicly by the military but reflecting the feeling of a lot of other true-born Britons as well – was one of the factors which delayed the Chunnel for another century. It came to fruition only in the 1980s, and even then was delayed by Mrs Thatcher's insistence that it be financed by private capital – part of a delaying tactic by someone who would have preferred a road bridge.

Even then, dealing successfully with reluctant bankers and with contractors who had hoped to make a killing required the talents of an extraordinary figure, Sir Alistair Morton, a determined, some would say bloody-minded, South African-born industrialist and banker who would have been perfectly at home in the nineteenth century. In the event the Chunnel is opening only about a year late – the much-publicized delays appear marginal compared with the hesitations of the preceding century.

The opening exposed a painful contrast between French and British policy towards railways. The French had built a special new line, the TGV-Nord, capable of whisking trains the 326 km (204 miles) from the Chunnel to Paris in 86 minutes, an average speed of (228 kph) (143 mph). In contrast the British government had allowed British Rail only enough money to patch up a route from the Chunnel to London using existing lines, often crowded with commuter traffic, and permitting an average speed of a mere 64 mph (102 kph), and even slower in the crucial rush hours. The government dodged the need for a new route by pretending, against all the evidence, that it could be privately financed.

The TGV-Nord is merely the latest in a series of new lines, and not only in France, which provided clear evidence of the return of the train from outer darkness. To do so required, if not a quantum leap in terms of speed, at least a major acceleration of a process which had gone on for 150 years until 1939, but which lost momentum until the 1970s.

For trains to compete with aeroplanes they had to speed up, though not, over a lot of routes, to an unimaginable extent. The rough rule of thumb is that trains are competitive with aeroplanes only for journeys of less than three hours. The best of orthodox trains are competitive only for distances of 250–300 miles (400–480 km) – like those from New York to Washington or London to Manchester – though electrification of the east coast route has meant that Newcastle, 273 miles (440 km) from London, is now comfortably within the 'three-hour circle'. But, obviously, increasing speeds to 150 or 200 mph (240 or 320 kph) increased the number of possible connections exponentially – and ensured the viability of the new lines, as long as they connected major conurbations. Hence it is relatively easy to predict which routes have the potential for new lines.

Throughout railway history speeds had increased only in fits and starts. The first record was set by George Stephenson himself when he reached 36 mph (58 kph) in carrying the body of William Huskisson to hospital. This was an exceptional run, as were many of the other records claimed over the next century and a half, from the first mile-a-minute run (by the GWR in 1845) to the first time a locomotive had achieved 100 mph (160 kph) – by the New York Central and the GWR at the turn of the century – to the 126 mph (203 kph) of the steam engine *Mallard* in 1938 and the 133.5 mph (215 kph) attained by the diesel-powered *Flying Hamburger* the following year.

More significant were the average speeds achieved on regular services, though even these were usually achieved by trains which were special, and thus irregular and more expensive. The intermittent nature of the speeding-up process can best be seen on Brunel's original line from London to Bristol and then on to Exeter. In the 1840s trains were already averaging over 40 mph (65 kph) and few, if any, regular services anywhere in the world averaged more than 50 mph (80 kph) in the next seventy years. Indeed the time required to travel the 120 miles (195 km) between London and Bristol was a mere 2 hours 45 minutes by 1852. It took another fifty years to reduce the time to 2 hours and another seventy to bring it down to 1 hour 30 minutes.

France's TGV seemingly disturbs neither cattle nor even Cluny, one of Burgundy's most famous abbeys.

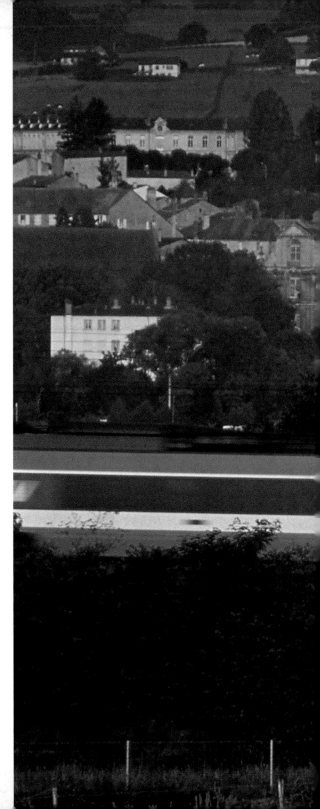

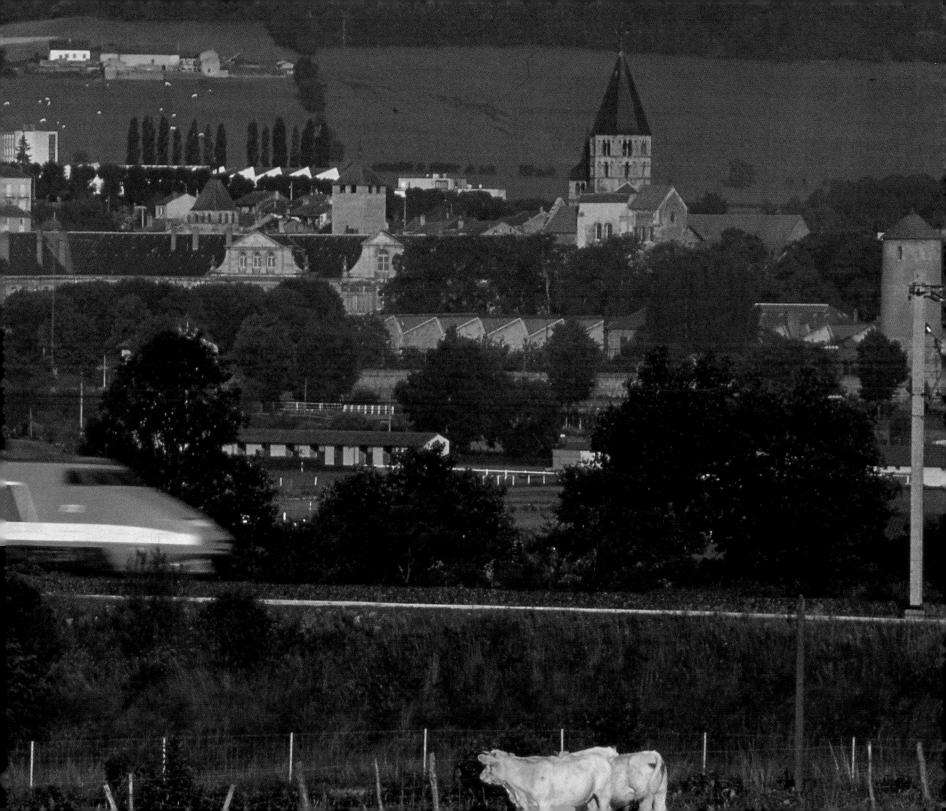

It was only between the wars that a handful of services started to average a mile a minute (97 kph) over any considerable distances. In the 1930s runs of over 70 mph (113 kph) were achieved by a number of steam-driven expresses in Britain like the Cheltenham Flyer with an average of 81.6 mph (131.3 kph) and by the exciting breed of streamlined trains powered by diesel-electric engines in the United States, trains like the Burlington Zephyr, which in the late 1930s averaged an amazing 77 mph (124 kph) on runs of up to nearly a thousand miles. The war put a stop to any such attempts, and, in the United States, speeds have still never recovered to anything like their pre-war levels. Elsewhere, inevitably, given the nature of railways, jumps in speed have depended on new trains (the diesel-powered High Speed Train was responsible for the speeding up of the old GWR service) or awaited a complete reconstruction or electrification of a line, as happened in France in the three decades after the war and in Britain when the line from London to Crewe was electrified in the 1960s, resulting in trains averaging 80 mph (130 kph).

Spain's first ultra-fast line was built in record time to take passengers from Madrid to Expo 92 in Seville.

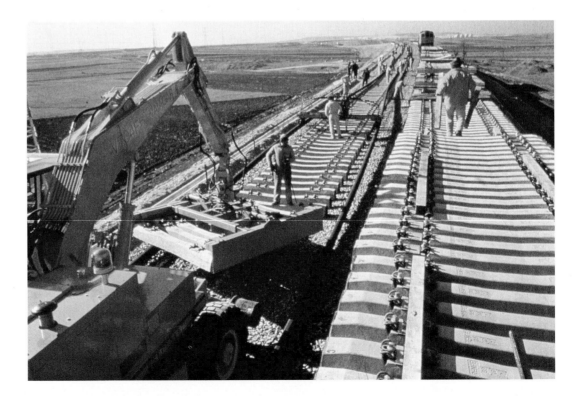

The event which marks the start of the railways' comeback as a modern form of passenger transport did not, in fact, use trains travelling at an inordinate speed – the average was only 160 kph (100 mph), 32 kph (20 mph) more than BR's trains, which were running on tracks laid down in the 1830s and 1840s. Nevertheless, 1 October 1964, when the Japanese National Railways opened their new line between Tokyo and Osaka, remains a crucial date in railway history. The Shinkansen, as it is popularly known (meaning 'new train': the line's official title, the Tokaido line, means simply 'Route Number One'), was not only a pioneering line but also the first symbol of Japan's industrial renaissance. It demonstrated clearly that the Japanese would no longer be confined to imitating others but would lead the world, and restated the original perception of railways as the prime symbol of national technical prowess.

In the quarter of a century since the opening of the new line the Japanese have been joined by the French, the Italians, the Germans and the Spanish, and new lines are being built, or at least planned, in countries as far apart as Korea, Switzerland and the United States. To build a new line has become – as it was a hundred and fifty years ago – a symbol that a country is serious in its efforts to show itself advanced and modern.

The route between Tokyo and Osaka was an ideal laboratory for fast trains: two-fifths of the country's population, and three-quarters of the nation's factories, were concentrated on the 2 per cent of land forming the narrow strip between the mountains and the sea. The Japanese had been planning the new route only since 1957, and in 1959 they decided to go ahead with the new line on the historic Western gauge (previous lines had been narrower) and to use 25,000 volt alternating current, already adopted by British Rail for its electrification of the line from London to Birmingham, Manchester and Glasgow. This posed technical problems. Like so much in railway history, it was an evolutionary, not a revolutionary advance on previous systems (which usually used the less efficient direct current, at lower voltages, either 750 or 1500 volts).

From the start the Shinkansen was a wild success, and within ten years was carrying a million passengers every day. Since 1964 the Japanese have extended their ultra-fast lines – though not as far as they had first dreamed – and increased the average speeds to around 225 kph (140 mph).

The Shinkansen acted as a challenge for other dreamers of railway improvements who had not previously dared to utter their thoughts in public (or felt they would not be taken seriously in the decade of the all-conquering motor car).

It also set two other crucial precedents: it provided a regular service and democratized speed, for the fares were no greater than on ordinary trains. The Japanese had also anticipated another trend, pioneered in Europe by British Rail: the idea that fast trains were no longer special but were simply part of a regular, often an hourly service. The British name Intercity soon came to indicate the idea of regular fast trains, not the occasional specials or 'Limiteds' which had been the historical norm.

Prior to what the Japanese might have termed the Shinkansen-shoku, the French had followed the same route as most countries. Over 20,000 km (12,500 miles) of lines had been abandoned (far more than in Britain, though with less fuss). After the war many lines had been electrified and in 1955 the French ran a special train at 331 kph (206 mph). Unfortunately the engine burnt out and the locomotives were mounted on such heavy and inflexible bogies that the track had to be completely renewed. But there were no new lines; indeed the last one (between Nice and Coni) had been opened in 1928 and the opening of a mere 2.5 km (1.5 miles) of new track in 1974 in the Paris suburbs was hailed as a major achievement.

But within a year of the opening of the new Tokaido line the French had produced the first draft of a plan for what was immediately named the TGV, the Train à Grande Vitesse, which envisaged a maximum speed of 320 kph (200 mph) and an average speed of 215–240 kph (135–150 mph). Although the first studies were conducted by the Northern region – and the first TGV could have been built between Paris and the Channel if the plans for a Chunnel had borne fruit in the 1970s – the obvious priority for a new line was the heavily-used route between Paris and Lyon, which echoed the parameters of the original Tokaido line. Moreover the existing line was a dogleg of 512 km (320 miles), and it soon proved practicable to use a direct route of a mere 425 km (266 miles). This could take advantage of the virtually unlimited power available from electric traction, allowing the line to have unprecedentedly steep gradients.

By the time the line was opened in the early 1980s the distance could be covered in

Opposite *The Bullet Train penetrates into the Ginza, in the heart of Tokyo.*

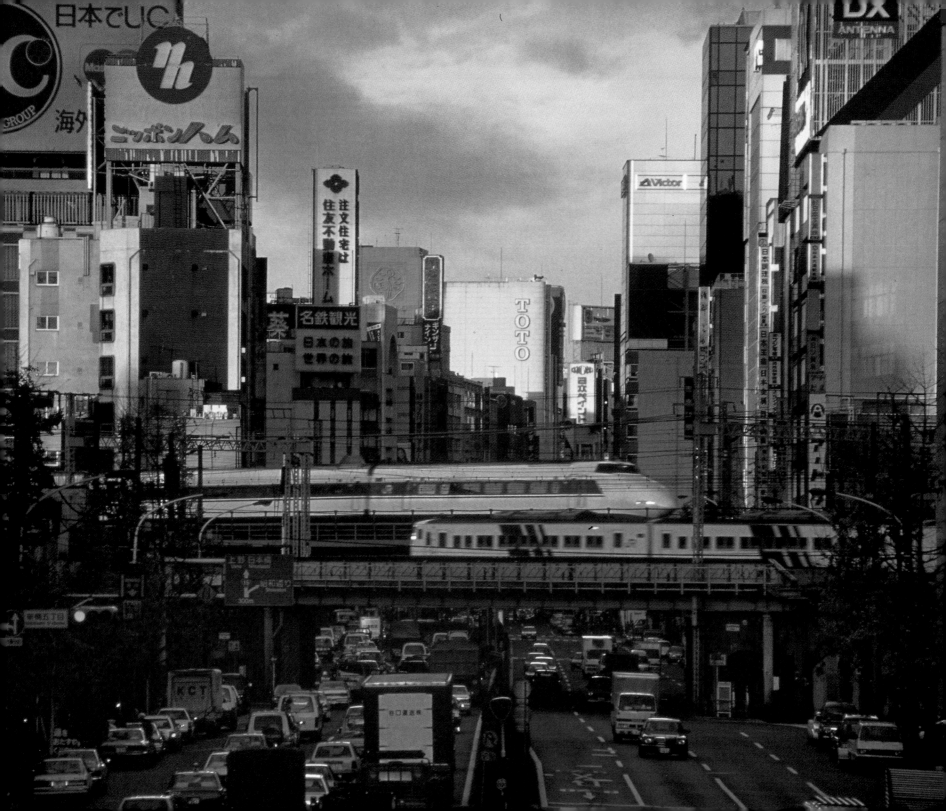

2 hours (as against 3 hours 47 minutes by a single special service, the Mistral, in pre-TGV days). The only radically new technology employed was in the signalling. Like the Shinkansen, the TGV was too fast for orthodox line-side signals so communication had to be by radio. The French also reduced the cost by using 19 km (12 miles) of existing tracks out of the Gare de Lyon in Paris and a further few kilometres on the last stretch into Lyon without too much loss of time.

The project faced numerous delays. Some were political, although it was finally given the green light in 1973 partly because the then head of the SNCF was a friend of the President, Georges Pompidou. The main political problem was that Dijon, capital of Burgundy, was to be bypassed. In the end a branch of the TGV was built directly to the city, served by ten special TGVs daily.

In the event, despite strikes and a series of uncommonly rainy summers, the TGV opened on time in October 1981. This was thanks partly to the SNCF's ability to rely on the sheer central power of the French state, but also the tact of the executives involved. The whole project was in the hands of a Polytechnician, Paul Avenas, an SNCF veteran who had already been in charge of the electrification of the old line from Paris to Lyon.

Inevitably the cost trebled between the first plan at the end of the 1960s and the opening. This was partly the effect of inflation and partly the cost of electrification: until the oil price rise of 1973 the TGV was to be powered by gas turbines.

As had happened so often in the nineteenth century, the traffic forecasts proved far too conservative. In 1976 the planners had foreseen 12.26 million passengers using the line every year, 68 per cent from the existing line, a mere 8 per cent motorists, and the remaining quarter from the airlines. The SNCF owned a quarter of Air Inter, which provided most of France's domestic air services, and in the 1980s the Lyon airport was moved to a new site 48 km (30 miles) from the centre of the city.

The SNCF was also happily surprised by the way so many passengers braved the 'three-hour barrier', using trains which ran only part of the time on the new tracks. They preferred to spend 3 hours 20 minutes to travel from Paris to Geneva by train or 4 hours 30 minutes from Paris to Marseilles rather than take the plane.

The success of the TGV-Sud Est, as it was termed, led to pressure from every other

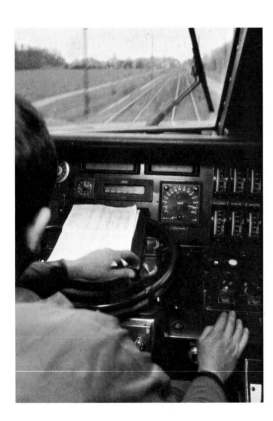

*All is calm in the cab
of the record-breaking TGV
as it accelerates towards
500 kph (310 mph).*

French region for a TGV of its own. Next on the agenda was the TGV-Atlantique, serving both Brittany and the South West. Here the SNCF was lucky: it discovered an unused suburban line which ran to within 6 kilometres of the TGV's Paris terminus at the Gare Montparnasse. By the time the line opened in 1991 the SNCF had improved the trains, as the suspension of the original TGVs had proved too hard for the older tracks on which it ran south of Lyon and east of Dijon. Fears about the ability of the train to cope with higher speeds had proved unjustified, and the biggest problem was the ability of the pantograph on top of the engine to capture current at over 320 kph (200 mph).

The pressure for new services continues. Bordeaux is furious that the original plans for the southward march of the TGV-Aquitaine did not pass directly through the city, and when the route of the third new line, the TGV-Nord to Brussels with a branch to the Channel Tunnel, was being traced, it was deemed essential that it pass through Lille, the stronghold of Pierre Mauroy, one of the leaders of the ruling Socialist party. Despite loud objections, Amiens, smaller and with less political clout, was bypassed, although it will be on the future line direct from Paris to the Chunnel.

By the end of the 1980s, the SNCF's plans were meeting some resistance. Any environmental objections to the earlier TGVs had been swamped by the gratitude of recipients of the new services. But the SNCF went too far in its plans to extend the original TGV further south. The route round Lyon to Valence was built without a murmur, but plans for the route further down the Rhône valley and through Provence to Marseilles, with a branch to Nice, proved that there was a limit, albeit a far-distant one, to the TGV, and thus, by implication, to fast routes as a whole.

The opposition included every possible lobby, from viticulturalists to lovers of Roman ruins and of the scenery round Mont Ste Victoire, the mountain overlooking Aix-en-Provence which had been Cézanne's favourite subject. The opposition also raised two key points: was not the SNCF being rather greedy in trying to compete with air travel on the route from Paris to Nice, 900 km (560 miles) away, and could not the new tracks follow the old on the way to Marseilles? The argument also raised another point: were not the French getting rather megalomaniac in hoping to make Paris into the centre of a new European high-speed network?

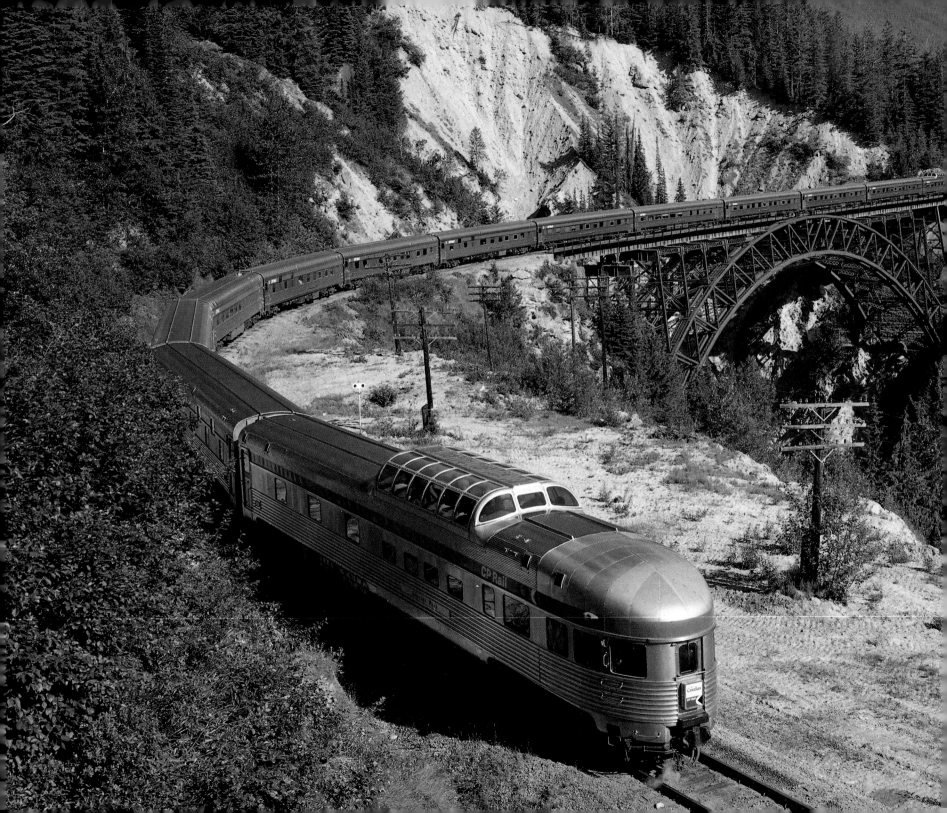

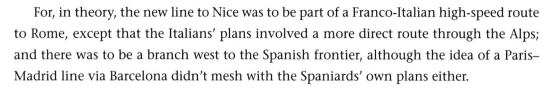

For, in theory, the new line to Nice was to be part of a Franco-Italian high-speed route to Rome, except that the Italians' plans involved a more direct route through the Alps; and there was to be a branch west to the Spanish frontier, although the idea of a Paris–Madrid line via Barcelona didn't mesh with the Spaniards' own plans either.

Spain was only one of the countries which have followed the French example. The most obvious case is the Germans. They have had to adapt their original plans. Their first high-speed line, from Hamburg south to Munich, was designed to counteract the fact that the existing network tended to run east–west – in other words to and from Berlin. The West German government's plans were drawn up on the assumption that the Iron Curtain was permanent, and that they would not have ready access to their former capital in the foreseeable future. They were also handicapped by the strength of regional governments and of ecological feeling, which greatly increased the cost of introducing new tracks in urban areas – and delayed for decades a new route on the most crowded of all lines, along the Rhine between Frankfurt and Cologne.

The direction of their efforts had to be completely changed when the two Germanys were reunited in 1990. This involved the highly expensive reconstruction of the ageing route network in the former East Germany, but, in the longer run, it provided Germany, or rather Berlin, with the opportunity for becoming the transport capital of Europe, since it is the natural centre for rail traffic between Russia, Poland and the west, and for traffic from Scandinavia, running through the new tunnels and bridges from Sweden and Denmark, to southern Europe. So the next decade could see a renewal of the old imperial battles of a century earlier, with the French and Germans using railways as weapons. The Germans are already competing with the French for the world speed record, which was held for a few months by the Germans' ICE train, until it was recaptured by the French in 1992 when a largely unmodified TGV reached a speed of over 480 kph (300 mph).

But other countries have their own plans. The Italians dreamed early, but ineffectually. The *Direttissima*, to run down the peninsula all the way from Milan and Turin to Bologna,

One of the regrettably rare trains which allow Canadians to appreciate the glories of their country's landscape.

Florence, Rome and Naples, was first put forward in Mussolini's days, in 1934. But progress has been episodic, if that, and only in late 1992 – after most of the work on the Rome–Florence line had been completed – did the authorities give the go-ahead to the whole project.

The Spaniards provided a complete contrast, building a totally new line between Madrid and Seville in time for the 1992 Exhibition. This line was largely political, to help the impoverished southern province of Andalucia, since it was uneconomic, with no prospect of any connection with the rest of the Spanish network – it was built on the normal European gauge, although all the other Spanish trains run on a 1675 cm (5 ft 6 in) gauge – and plans for the most sensible new line, between Madrid and Barcelona, are still not well advanced.

The trend has spread to such aspirants to 'truly-advanced' status as Korea, Taiwan and Turkey. The line the Turks are building from Istanbul to the capital Ankara shows just how backward rail transport had become and how the most obvious linkages had been neglected, to the great advantage of road transport. At the moment the roundabout trip takes over seven hours. On the new line trains will take $2\frac{1}{2}$ hours, running at 172 kph (107 mph), a pretty conservative timing for a new line, and barely faster than BR's trains to Newcastle along a line of similar length completed in the early 1850s. But perhaps the most defiant gesture is being made by the Russians who have formed a joint company to build a new line covering the 657 km (408 miles) between Moscow and St Petersburg – an ideal length for a new line.

But it is the Swiss who have gone the furthest in the return journey to the train. Not only are they pressing ahead with their Alpine tunnels, and with new lines, they also have a clear national policy called Bahn 2000. Their first idea is to remove heavy lorries – especially those passing through – from their roads, a priority they share with the Austrians, who are already rationing the number of lorries which can travel over the Brenner pass. But, even more ambitiously, they are putting the final touches on the world's most elaborate plan for passenger rail services. This involves a timetable which ensures that trains leave major urban centres precisely on the hour and the half-hour.

Unfortunately, the Swiss project is proving far more expensive than planned, partly because the environmental lobby is so strong that even the short stretches of new line required are meeting unforeseen opposition. But, despite delays, the plans remain firm, and in the early years of the twenty-first century the country could enjoy an incomparable rail service.

*A*merican plans for high-speed passenger trains are still in the embryonic stage but Amtrak, the publicly-owned long-distance passenger rail system, has come a long way since the early 1980s when David Stockman, then President Reagan's Budget Director, stormed against any further help, claiming that it was neither a necessary nor important part of the national transportation system – a 'mobile money-burning machine', in the words of one of its critics, serving less than 1 per cent of the country's intercity travellers.

But, after a twenty-year fight to preserve any sort of passenger service even the Americans are coming to realize the railways' value in passenger transport. The battle has been bitter. In 1971, when Amtrak was formed, President Nixon would have preferred to abandon the whole idea, but eventually funds were found for a basic publicly-owned passenger service. The biggest single step came in 1976 when Amtrak bought the track between New York and Washington from the then-nationalized Conrail system. This has enabled Amtrak to provide regular services between the two cities which now take 40 per cent of the traffic on what is known as the North-East Corridor.

But on its long-distance routes Amtrak has never been able to run more than a skeletal service, with trains running at most twice daily and often only a couple of times a week. Many are openly tourist trains bearing nostalgic names – the Desert Wind from Chicago to Los Angeles, and the Empire Builder from Chicago to Seattle. These services are often booked solid in the summer months by tourists anxious to see some of the country's most inspiring scenery from the comfort of sleeping and dining cars.

Amtrak has always suffered from severe constraints. Many of its carriages are still what it calls 'heritage' stock, inherited from other railroads when it was formed, average speeds rarely reach more than 50 mph (80 kph) and its reliability record is poor. This is because (apart from the North-East Corridor) Amtrak is running passenger trains on lines

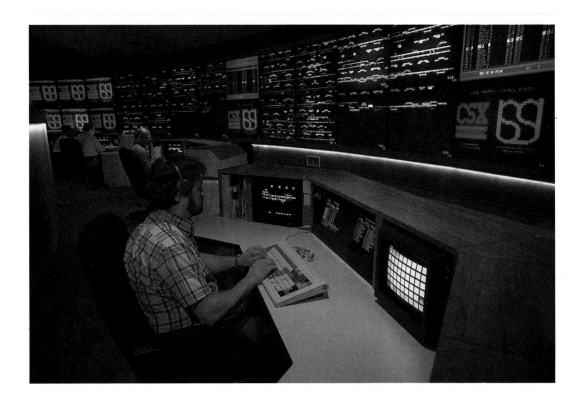

CSX's control centre at Jacksonville in Florida looks as though it is tracking a space shuttle rather than the trains on its 19,000 miles (30,570 kms) of railway track.

normally used by relatively slow freight trains whose timings are less exact. So although nine out of ten passenger trains on Amtrak's own route from Washington to New York are on time, the figure falls below two thirds elsewhere.

Amtrak was lucky that during the Reagan years it had as its chairman Graham Claytor, the sort of lawyer cum public servant symbolized by men like Dean Acheson. Claytor, for twenty years a partner in Acheson's law firm, was the last of the old-style 'wise men', a former Secretary of the Navy, and more relevantly, a former chairman of the Southern Railroad – one of the country's most efficient. It was his sheer love of railroads, and a sense of public duty, which led him to take on the Amtrak job in 1982 when he was already seventy years old.

By a natural sense of thrift and dogged attention to detail he steadily improved Amtrak's services, and, more crucially, its finances. Between 1981 and 1988 revenue increased by 30 per cent in real terms and by 1988 Amtrak was covering 69 per cent of its costs, against a mere 48 per cent seven years earlier. Claytor also grasped at every other commercial possibility open to him, whether it was property, laying fibre optic cables alongside the rails, mail handling or collecting fees from operating commuter train services. A further victory in 1991 ensured that the government took on Amtrak's pension obligations and thus improved the operating ratio still further.

The public mood started to change under President Bush, and Claytor was able to claw in some crucial funds to renew Amtrak's ageing locomotives and rolling stock – the average age of which was a startling $21\frac{1}{2}$ years. More promisingly, the Bush administration identified five 'corridors' possibly suitable for long-term investment.

Under Claytor Amtrak's ambitions have remained modest. Even his presentation to Congress on services 'to areas not presently served' implied only modest improvements with incremental subsidies of a few million dollars to achieve such worth-while, but limited objectives as the extension of the Chicago-Milwaukee service to Green Bay.

But before he retired in the summer of 1993, universally hailed as the saviour of the country's rail passenger system, he did set in motion a major extension of the North-East corridor from New York to Boston, a journey of a mere 230 miles (371 km) which now takes a full five hours. By 1997 electrification, some modest track improvements – and the purchase of tilting trains from the Swedes – could reduce the journey to well below the crucial three-hour mark, but even this would represent an average speed of below the 80 mph (129 kph) reached today by the Metroliners running from Washington to New York. Elsewhere a variety of pressure groups are working on much more ambitious plans. These include a handful of truly ultra-fast lines in obvious corridors: plans are furthest advanced for the route between Houston, San Antonio and Fort Worth in Texas. But possibly the most encouraging feature of the scene is the renewed interest by state and municipal governments in passenger railways. Even more ambitious are the plans put forward by the leading crusader for supertrains, Joseph Vranich, author of an influential book of the same name. But there are still many battles to be fought before any of these plans actually produce concrete results.

By contrast, the United States has been at the forefront of the other revolution of the 1980s, the belated attempt by railways the world over to compete with trucks for freight traffic. This is partly because of the nature of the country: for obvious reasons rail transport is not competitive with road traffic for short hauls below 200–300 miles (300–450 km).

In Europe the fight has been half-hearted, at best. At its worst, a short-sighted British government had forced British Rail to charge such vast sums for use of its tracks that one promising service, Charterrail, which used specially adapted road trailers, was forced off the rails by excessive track charges. And, even though other European rail authorities have received backing from their governments, a combination of bureaucratic inertia and the inability of the railway authorities to work together have prevented any real shift of freight off the roads – especially as truckers are being forced to charge prices far lower than they need to replace their trucks.

The situation is very different in the United States, where, finally, Congress has admitted that the railways are not an over-mighty force requiring tight controls. In 1976 the 'Four R' Act removed the fear of anti-trust suits, and since the Staggers Act was passed in 1980 the railroads have undergone a revolution. The change was at the last minute: 'without deregulation the system would have collapsed with the depression of the early 1980s', says the veteran railroad analyst, Henry Livingston of Kidder Peabody. He was not exaggerating. In one famous case the merger of the Rock Island line with the Union Pacific was held up for eleven long years by a series of anti-trust suits. By the time they were settled the Rock Island was bankrupt and the Union Pacific no longer interested.

So when the Staggers Act finally freed the railroads after nearly a century of increasingly tight restrictions only a certified madman would have forecast a comeback so triumphant that within little more than a decade railroad stocks would be more highly valued than those of the country's airlines. But such was the case.

First came concentration. Within a few years the bulk of the nation's railroad mileage was in the hands of only six systems: CSX, Conrail and Norfolk & Southern in the east, south and mid-west, Burlington Northern across the north and north-west, and in the west and south-west the Union Pacific, Santa Fe and Southern Pacific – and even these last two would like to have merged, a move blocked by the otherwise-inactive Interstate Commerce Commission.

The public finally woke up to the railroads' renaissance in 1985 when Ms Elizabeth

Dole, then Secretary for Transport, tried to sell Conrail to Norfolk & Southern for a mere $1.2 billion, far less than the $7 billion the taxpayer had poured into the bankrupt system since it had been nationalized in 1976. After a major outcry, Conrail was successfully floated on Wall Street at a far higher value, and neither the stock nor the system has looked back since. An even greater tribute has come from the major long-distance truck companies who, increasingly, are using railroads for long hauls.

Truckers and railroads alike are fighting a defensive war against general economic trends. At the end of the decade the railroads were actually carrying less freight than in 1980 – and coal, their core business, still accounts for near two-fifths of their total. Elsewhere the general shift away from older heavy industries – like steel and bulk chemicals – the railroads' staple diet over the past century, has reduced the total traffic available. Increased imports have dealt a double blow where, as with iron and steel, the railroads relied on transporting the raw materials as well as the finished products. Other key customers, like the motor manufacturers, had become accustomed to 'just-in-time' service from truckers, so had to be wooed back with costly guarantees of a reliability they had not enjoyed from the railroads for a generation or more. And competition, from heavily-subsidized water transport as well as from the truckers, meant that freight rates declined steadily throughout the 1980s.

But the railroads flourished, for the new freedom unleashed an unsuspected, and long-suppressed capacity for greater efficiency and better management, backed by massive investment. During the 1980s they poured over $30 billion into track and signals and another $100 billion into maintenance. They also found the money for technical innovations, a thing of the distant past: improvements in the design of wheels (literally 'reinventing the wheel') saved the railroads over $100 million annually in repair bills.

Perhaps the greatest improvement came in the management of their assets, notably their wagons, vastly increasing the mileage they ran, while at the same time reducing claims from their customers for damage and late deliveries by nearly $200 million annually. Better equipment and more care meant that the accident rate dropped by over half.

During the decade the railroads succeeded in securing much of the 'intermodal'

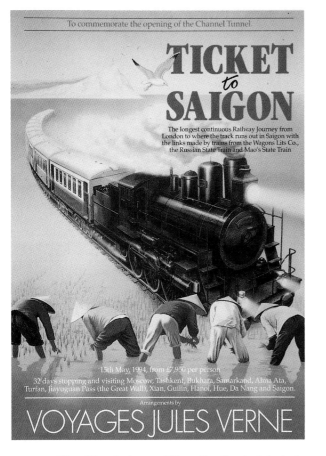

To commemorate the opening of the Channel Tunnel.

TICKET *to* SAIGON

The longest continuous Railway Journey from London to where the track runs out in Saigon with the links made by trains from the Wagons Lits Co., the Russian State Train and Mao's State Train

15th May, 1994, from £7,950 per person

32 days stopping and visiting Moscow, Tashkent, Bukhara, Samarkand, Alma Ata, Turfan, Jiayuguan Pass (the Great Wall), Xian, Guilin, Hanoi, Hue, Da Nang and Saigon.

Arrangements by

VOYAGES JULES VERNE

The ultimate dream of the rail enthusiast: by train direct from Moscow to Saigon.

business, double-stacking containers to transport imported goods from the Far East from Pacific ports to America's heartland. The Norfolk & Southern went further, experimenting with RoadRailers, equipped with both rubber tyres (for use on roads) and steel wheels for use on railroad tracks. These were far more efficient than containers, which required a structural underframe to be transportable by rail. Other, initially sceptical, railroads are now following Norfolk & Southern's example.

They are also following CSX and Union Pacific, which have installed elaborate centralized control systems, enabling the bosses to know exactly where every train (and soon every wagon) in their fleet is at any moment. The system – like the railroads themselves – are still run largely by executives brought up on the old regulated days, a striking tribute to the adaptability of men usually dismissed as inflexible.

CSX's control centre looks like an air traffic control room, for railroads are not too proud to learn from their rivals. The chairman of Burlington Northern, Gerald Grinstein, is a former airline executive and has introduced one of their key ideas, the 'launch order' for a new piece of equipment, in this case new AC diesel-electric locomotives. By placing an order for 150 of these monsters, he is saving his railroad over $500,000 a locomotive, and ensuring that it is equipped with the latest machines well before any of its rivals.

Railroads have even successfully tackled their greatest problem: a bloated, overpaid, well-organized workforce. Hundreds of thousands of jobs had been lost in the decade before Staggers, but in the 1980s numbers were halved again to under 250,000, although wages remained far above the national industrial average and not all restrictive practices were removed (it was only after a series of battles that the 'normal' working day for train crews was redefined as more than a hundred miles – it is still only 130 (209 km), a mere couple of hours journey for an intermodal express.)

Part of the improvement sprang from a concentration of business: first on the most important customers – nine-tenths of CSX's business comes from one hundred companies – and then by chopping unwanted lines. In the 1980s, helped by a court decision which made the process far easier, the major railroads eliminated 41,000 miles (66,000 km) of track. Many of these simply duplicated other routes (the railroad map of the United States shows just how many more could be abandoned without any threat to services between major centres) but others served towns and customers too small to be of economic interest to a big organization.

A great many of these routes were taken up by a new breed of entrepreneurs, the 'short-line operators' transporting everything from china clay in Georgia to wine in California. The revolution is also social: 'our primary focus is small-town America', says William Loftus, President of the American Short Line Railroad Association, whose membership has nearly doubled in the past fifteen years.

Despite the growing opportunities as the major Class One railroads divest themselves of track and customers the short lines face a major problem: improving their equipment. They usually inherited old and aged track, nearly half of it dating from before the 1930s when a new type of rail was introduced which greatly reduced breakages. Not surprisingly trains are limited to below 25 mph (40 kph) on over half the 24,600 miles (40,000 km) of track owned by Loftus' members, and they can run at over 40 mph (64 kph) on only 3000 miles (4800 km).

But the shortliners are typical entrepreneurs, unafraid of the future – while still lobbying hard for help in renewing their tracks, for they are reverting to the primal type which created the railroads in the first place. In the words of Bruce Flohr, Chairman of RailTex which runs a number of unconnected short lines: 'We all like small a lot better. Most of us came from big companies. We're thriving on the small-company focus.' But, despite this resurgence of primitive capitalism, most railway initiatives elsewhere in the world remain in the hands of governments.

At last. After over a century of delays the first train emerges from the Chunnel – even though it had to be towed.

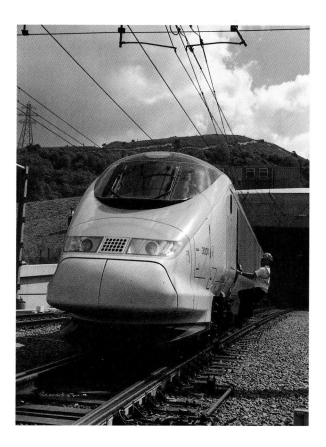

*T*he most spectacular new lines are relatively unknown, largely because they are mostly in Russia and China. As so often in the past, these were decided by geo-political factors. During the decades when the Soviet Union's relations with its Communist 'brothers' in China were as bad as with the capitalist West the Russians naturally tried to build a new variant for the eastern end of the Trans-Siberian, further away from the Chinese frontier. Although this, the so-called BAM, was also designed to tap the enormous reserves of coal and other minerals to the north of Lake Baikal, there is no doubt that, like the Trans-Siberian itself, it would not have been built without some additional geo-political, imperial impetus. Not unexpectedly, construction posed enormous problems, what with permafrost, bogs, marshes, and all the horrors of northern Siberian conditions. Worst of all was the need to build a 14-km (9-mile) tunnel at Severo-Muysk, to the north-east of Lake Baikal. This is in one of the world's worst seismic trouble spots, with up to 2500 tremors every year, resulting in continuing problems. But the Russians surmounted them all.

But, once the relationship between the two Communist super-powers had warmed, the Russians and the Chinese worked together to provide better links between Europe and the Pacific, in the hope of attracting traffic to the 'land-bridge' which, in theory, at least, provided a faster link between Europe and Japan and the Far East.

For railways remain a political instrument. In the middle of 1992 the Iranian President, Hashemi Rafsanjani, formally inaugurated construction of a long-planned line from Mashad to the border with Turkmenistan, thus providing an all-Muslim rail link to the Persian Gulf for the Muslim republics of Central Asia, which previously had to rely on rail links through Moscow and had no direct links to the sea. They are thus declaring their independence of the Russians in the same way as the Belgians declared their freedom from the Dutch over a hundred and sixty years earlier.

Hence the least-publicized and most fascinating new route of all. This runs south of Moscow, via Kubyshev and Tselingrad, into China's Wild West along a newly-built line over the unimaginably distant Alataw pass and thence through China to Shanghai. With the completion of the Channel Tunnel, this would provide a continuous rail route between, say, Liverpool and Shanghai. Who said railway dreams belonged to the nineteenth century?

Bibliography

General

Andrews, C. B., *The railway age*, Country Life, 1937. op.
Barman, C., *An introduction to railway architecture*, Art & Technics, 1950. op.
Bonavia, M. R. *The Channel Tunnel story*, David & Charles, 1987. op.
Carr, S., *The poetry of railways*, Batsford, 1978. op.
Ellis, C. H., *Railway art*, Ash & Grant, 1977. op.
Hobsbawm, E., *The age of capital, 1848–1875*, Weidenfeld & Nicolson, 1975; Cardinal, 1988. op.
Hobsbawm, E., *The age of empire, 1875–1914*, Weidenfeld & Nicolson, 1988; Cardinal, 1989.
Hopkins, K., *The poetry of railways: an anthology*, Frewin, 1966. op.
Huntley, J., *The Railways on the screen*, rev. edn. (of *The Railway in the Cinema*, 1969. op.) I. Allen, 1993.
Kennedy, L., *A book of railway journeys*, Collins, 1980; Fontana, 1981. op.
Mazlish, B., *The railroad and the space program: an exploration in historical analogy* U.S., MIT Press, 1965. op.
Meeks, C., *The railway station: an architectural history*, U.S., Architectural Press; Yale U.P., 1957. op.
Miller, C., *Lunatic express*, Macdonald, 1972; Futura, 1977. op.
O'Dell, A. C., *Railways and geography*, Hutchinson, 1971. op.
O'Brien, P., *The new economic history of the railways*, Croom Helm, 1977. op.
Richards, J. and MacKenzie, J. M., *The railway station: a social history*, Oxford U.P., 1988.
Robbins, M., *The railway age*, Routledge & Kegan Paul, 1962; Penguin, 1965. op.
Rolt, L. T. C., *Red for danger; a history of railway accidents and railway safety*, David & Charles, 4th edn., 1982, op.
Best railway stories, Faber, 1969. op.
Simmons, J. ed., *Railways: an anthology*, Collins, 1991. op.
Swinglehurst, E., *The romantic journey: the story of Thomas Cook and Victorian travel*, Pica Editions, 1974. op.
Theroux, P., *The great railway bazaar: by train through Asia*, Hodder, 1990; Penguin, 1977.
Van Creveld, M., *Supplying war: logistics from Wallenstein to Patton*, Cambridge U.P., 1977.

Britain

Barker, T. C. and Robbins, M., *History of London transport*. Vol 1: *Nineteenth century*, Allen & Unwin, 1963; 1975. op. Vol 2: *Twentieth century to 1970*, Allen & Unwin, 1976.
Biddle, G., *Great railway stations of Britain*, David & Charles, 1986. op.
Briggs, A., *Victorian cities*, Penguin, 1990.
Coleman, T., *The railway navvies: a history of the men who made railways*, Penguin, 1981.

Joby, R. S., *The railway builders: lives and works of the Victorian railway contractors*, David & Charles, 1983. op.
Kellett, J. R., *The impact of railways on Victorian cities*, Routledge & Kegan Paul, 1969. op.
Kingsford, P. W., *Victorian railwaymen: emergence and growth of railway labour, 1830–70*, P. Cass, 1970.
Lambert, R. S., *The railway king, 1800–1871: a study of George Hudson and the business morals of his time*, Allen & Unwin, 1964. op.
McKenna, F., *The railway workers, 1840–1970*, Faber, 1980. op.
Ransom, P. J. G., *The Victorian railway and how it evolved*, Heinemann, 1990. op.
Rolt, L. T. C. *Victorian engineering*, Allen Lane, 1970; Penguin, 1974. op.
Isambard Kingdom Brunel, Penguin, 1990.
George & Robert Stephenson: the railway revolution, Greenwood Press, 1977.
Simmons, J., *The railway in town and country, 1830–1914*, David & Charles, 1986. op.
The Victorian railway, Thames & Hudson, 1991.
Vaughan, A., *Isambard Kingdom Brunel: engineering knight errant*, J. Murray, 1991; pbk., 1993.
Walton, J. K., *The English seaside resort: a social history, 1750–1914*, Leicester U.P., 1983.

China

Han Suyin, *The crippled tree*, Panther, 1972.
Theroux, P., *Riding the iron rooster: by train through China*, H. Hamilton, 1988; Penguin, 1989.

France

Baroli, M., *Le train dans la litterature Française*, France, Vie du Rail, 1969.
Bazin, J. F., *Les defis du TGV*, France, Denoel, 1981.
O'Brien, P., *Railways and the economic development of Western Europe, 1830–1914*, Macmillan, 1983. op.
Weber, E., *Peasants into Frenchmen: the modernization of rural France*, Chatto Windus, 1977; pbk., 1979. op.

Latin America

Fawcett, B., *Railways of the Andes*, Allen & Unwin, 1963. op.
Kepner, C. D. Jr., *The banana empire: a case study of economic imperialism*, U.S., Russell & Russell, 1967. op.
Ross, D., *Visionaries & swindlers: the development of the railways of Honduras*, U.S., Institute for Research in Latin America, 1975. op.
Schott, J., *Rails across Panama*, U.S., Bobbs, 1967. op.
Stewart, W., *Henry Meiggs: Yankee Pizarro*, U.S., AMS Press, 1968. op.
Theroux, P., *The old Patagonian express: by train through the Americas*, Penguin, 1981.

North America

Abramson, R., *Spanning the century: the life of W. Averell Harriman, 1891–1986*, U.S., Morrow, 1992.
Beebe, L., *Mixed train daily: a book of short-line railroads*, U.S., Dutton; Smithers, 1947. op.
Berton, P., *The impossible railway: the building of the Canadian Pacific*, U.S., P. Smith, 1984.
Berton, P., *The promised land: settling the West, 1896–1914*, Canada, McClelland & Stewart, 1984. op.
Botkin, B. A. and Harlow, A. E., *A treasury of railroad folklore*, U.S., Outlet Book Co., 1989, repr. of 1953 edn.
Brown, D., *Hear that lonesome whistle blow: railroads in the west*, Chatto & Windus, 1977; Pan, 1979. op.
Calkins, E. E., *They broke the prairie*, Greenwood Press, 1971, repr. of 1937 edn.; U.S., University of Illinois Press, 1989.
Chandler, A., *Railroads: the nation's first big business: sources and readings*, U.S., Ayer, 1981.
The visible hand: the managerial revolution in American business, U.S., Belknap Press, 1977.
Henry Flagler: the astonishing life and times of the visionary robber baron who founded Florida, U.S., Macmillan, 1986.
Cohen, N., *Long steel rail: the railroad in American folksong*, U.S., Univeristy of Illinois Press, 1984.
Cummings, R. O., *The American and his food: a history of food habits in the United States*, U.S., Ayer, 1970. repr. of 1940 edn.
Douglas, G., *All aboard! The railroad in American life*, U.S., Paragon House, 1992.
Dunbar, S., *History of travel in America, Vol I*, U.S., Greenwood, 1968, repr. of 1915 edn.
Henderson, G. F. R., *Science of war*, U.S., Gordon Press, 1977.
Holbrook, S. H., *The story of American railroads*, U.S., Crown, 1982.
Josephson, M., *The robber barons: the great American capitalists, 1861–1901*, U.S., HarBrace, 1962.
Korson, G. G. ed., *Pennsylvania songs and legends*, U.S., Ayer, 1979.
Lewis, O., *The big four*, U.S., Ayer, 1981, repr. of 1938 edn.
Licht, W., *Working for the railroad*, U.S., Princeton UP, 1987.
Martin, A., *Railroads triumphant: the growth, rejection and rebirth of a vital American force*, U.S., Oxford UP, 1992.
Marx, L., *The machine in the garden: technology and the pastoral ideal in America*, U.S., Oxford U.P., 1964.
Stover, J. F., *Life and decline of the American railroad*, U.S., Oxford U.P., 1970. op.
Ward, J. A., *Railroads and the character of America, 1820–1887*, U.S., University of Tennessee Press, 1986.
Waters, L. L., *Steel trails to Santa Fe*, U.S., University of Kansas, 1950. op.
Williams, J. H., *A great and shining road: the epic story of the Transcontinental railroad*, U.S., Random, 1988.

Index